THE
CHALLENGE
JOURNAL

12 Proven Steps to Improve Mental Health

First published by Ultimate World Publishing 2024
Copyright © 2024 Katrina Langhorn

ISBN

Paperback: 978-1-923123-54-0
Ebook: 978-1-923123-55-7

Cover design: Ultimate World Publishing
Layout and typesetting: Ultimate World Publishing
Editor: Alex Floyd-Douglass

Ultimate World Publishing
Diamond Creek,
Victoria Australia 3089
www.writeabook.com.au

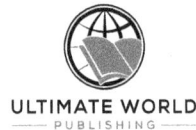

Dedication

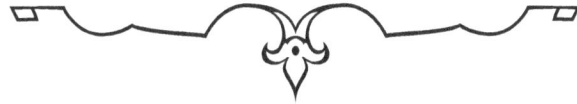

For my sons, William and David.

Disclaimer

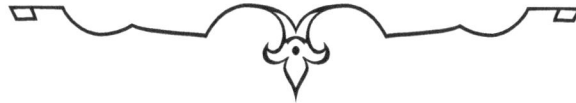

This book can offer support both before, during and after therapy. If you have experienced trauma, it is essential to seek professional advice.

The Australian Bureau of Statistics (2023) uses and supports the use of the Mindframe National Guidelines for responsible, accurate and safe reporting on mental health concerns. The guidelines were created to promote secure and precise reporting, representation, and communication of mental health issues. The goal is to diminish stigma and foster a willingness to seek help. It seeks to inform, support, and empower people to minimise stigma and harm.

In case of suicidal thoughts, please reach out to LIFELINE at 13 11 14, available 24/7 to provide help and support. I can verify this assistance, based on my experience volunteering for LIFELINE and the vital care they provide. If life is threatened, please call 000 or visit the closest Emergency Department.

This book serves as a tool – especially during extended waiting periods before the initial and between professional appointments. Remember to take this book with you, as it can facilitate your healthcare professional's understanding of your challenges and contribute to the therapeutic process.

No patient details have been used at all in this book. No animals have been harmed in the production of this book, unfortunately the same cannot be said

Testimonials

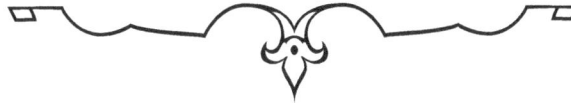

"Honestly, do yourself a favour and think about this book. Whether you are going through struggles, feel that you are stuck or even if you enjoy a fascinating read, I absolutely know that certain pages will resonate with everyone, even if to reassure that you are on the right path!"

Annie, Business Entrepreneur, Annie's Grazing Boxes

"The Challenge Journal is a comprehensive guide to self-determination, an adjunct to a clinician's practice enabling true growth for your clients. It demystifies counseling terms for the uninitiated. An excellent resource for clients and any allied health professional."

Wendy, Retired Nurse

"Over the years I have read many self-help books, however, Katrina's 'The Challenge Journal' goes beyond that by being a book on Self Awareness with many practical exercises.

It highlights many of life's challenges and gives you a positive way to act or react to various situations, giving a number of coping exercises as well as highlighting how to read the needs of others.

An easy read, with clearly defined chapters so you can pick it up at any chapter which you need at any particular time. I thoroughly recommend this work."

"Thoroughly researched and incredibly practical, this book is a must if you want to boost your engagement in enjoyable activities, enhance your social interactions, and alleviate psychological tension."

Emma, Psychologist

"Katrina Langhorn's, The Challenge Journal, is a 'survival manual' to help you live and appreciate the value of a better life. We all look to be filled up by something. Some want a lifestyle, others it is fame and glory, while another portion crave 'a knowing'.

I am one of the latter. Learning does it for me. Learning about what makes myself and others tick. Learning how to do better and be a wiser me. I have known depression intimately. To survive, I needed to learn how and counselling and education opened the way. The Challenge Journal will be on my bedside table until I master more. Thank you Katrina for sharing your insight and real-life tools to not just survive but thrive."

Brooke, Savvy Centric

"This is a practical guide with very easy to follow steps to change the way you live your life with others. Added to that, it has easy to understand phrases and clear definitions of more academic speak. This is a must read and a must act on purchase for people from every background."

Tina,
Therapist, The Blue Butterfly Institute Founder and Akashic Healing

Introduction

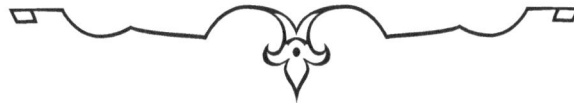

For over 20 years, I have worked as a psychologist in private practice helping thousands of patients, as well as working as an educator in many schools, including students in behavioural, disability and selective settings. In addition, I have presented nationally and facilitated many workshops on the topics included in this book.

I have worked in hospitals and forensic settings, including volunteering for *LIFELINE's* 24-hour crisis support and suicide prevention hotline, *Youth Off the Streets*, working with homeless youth and *Disability Services Australia*. I have also supervised provisional psychologists on their internships and mentored university students.

Without fail, in every session I have utilised one or more of the following tools and strategies listed in each of the chapters. The chapters in this book are designed to complement each other, but there is no strict requirement to read them sequentially.

If you find it more convenient to navigate based on your specific needs or interests, using the table of contents to locate relevant topics – it can be just as beneficial. If some parts seem overly heavy or confusing, don't give up. Try to just do some

This Challenge Journal predominantly utilises Cognitive Behavioural Therapy (CBT) techniques with the aim of boosting engagement in enjoyable activities, enhancing social interactions, refining conflict resolution and problem-solving abilities, alleviating physiological tension and excessive emotional arousal and recognising and altering attributions and beliefs associated with depressive thoughts.

This Challenge Journal also uses Acceptance and Commitment Therapy (ACT) approaches such as mindfulness practices, alongside Narrative Therapy. Acceptance and Commitment Therapy (ACT), mindfulness practices and Narrative Therapy are therapeutic approaches that can be integrated to create a comprehensive and effective treatment plan. Each approach brings its unique perspective and techniques to the therapeutic process.

This book's intention is hope.

*NB: Included in each chapter, you will find mindful pictures to colour in. In the back section of this book is a Psychology Dictionary – any word throughout the book with an * has a definition at the back. There is also a reference section if you would like to look something up and a HELP section for support organisations available to you.*

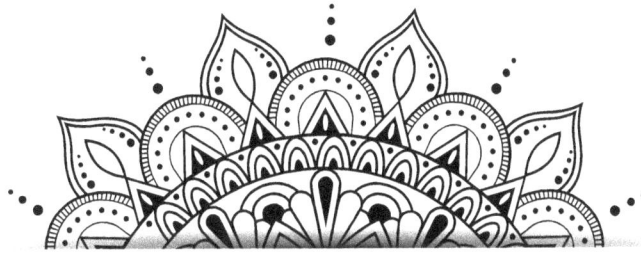

CHAPTER 1

Improve Your Communication

"The single biggest problem in communication is the illusion that it has taken place." (George Bernard Shaw)

Effective communication is the cornerstone of meaningful interactions, but what separates good communicators from the rest? In this chapter, we will explore the art of assertive communication. In my experience, good assertive communicators tend to enjoy several advantages:

- They convey their message accurately the first time and to the right people.
- They minimise misunderstandings.
- They build better relationships with their family, friends, and colleagues.
- They give the impression of confidence, have clear boundaries and are more likely to have their needs met.

According to a survey by Richardson (2022), more than half of the people reported

57% indicated that they have grown more assertive as they have aged, while 43% acknowledged the need to actively acquire assertiveness skills.

The good news is that we can all learn to be more assertive communicators; it's not rocket science. But first, we must understand the difference between passive, aggressive and assertive communication styles, so we know where on the continuum we are situated.

Communication; the dance of words and gestures. It's like a two-way street where information takes a scenic route from one mind to another.

On the passive side, it is like surrendering the stage, letting others take the spotlight while your needs take a back seat. It's a bit like saying, *"Oh, you go ahead, I'm just here for the ride."*

Then, on the aggressive side, it is like being the diva of communication, grabbing the microphone and drowning out everyone else. It's all about making sure your needs are front and centre, even if it means elbowing others out of the way.

Finding that sweet spot in the middle – assertive communication – is like hitting the communication bullseye. It's saying what you need to say without trampling on others or fading into the background. Striking that balance is an art that gets better with practice; the more you practice the better you will become.

I will often suggest to my clients to practice on their pet. Yes, you read that correctly! Our pets, especially dogs, tend to love us unconditionally and won't mind you practising your novice assertive communication style. As long as you're giving them attention, they are a willing audience.

❧ **Psych tip:** *Goldfish are not quite as helpful.*

Let's have a look at a picture diagram while we examine the different terms.

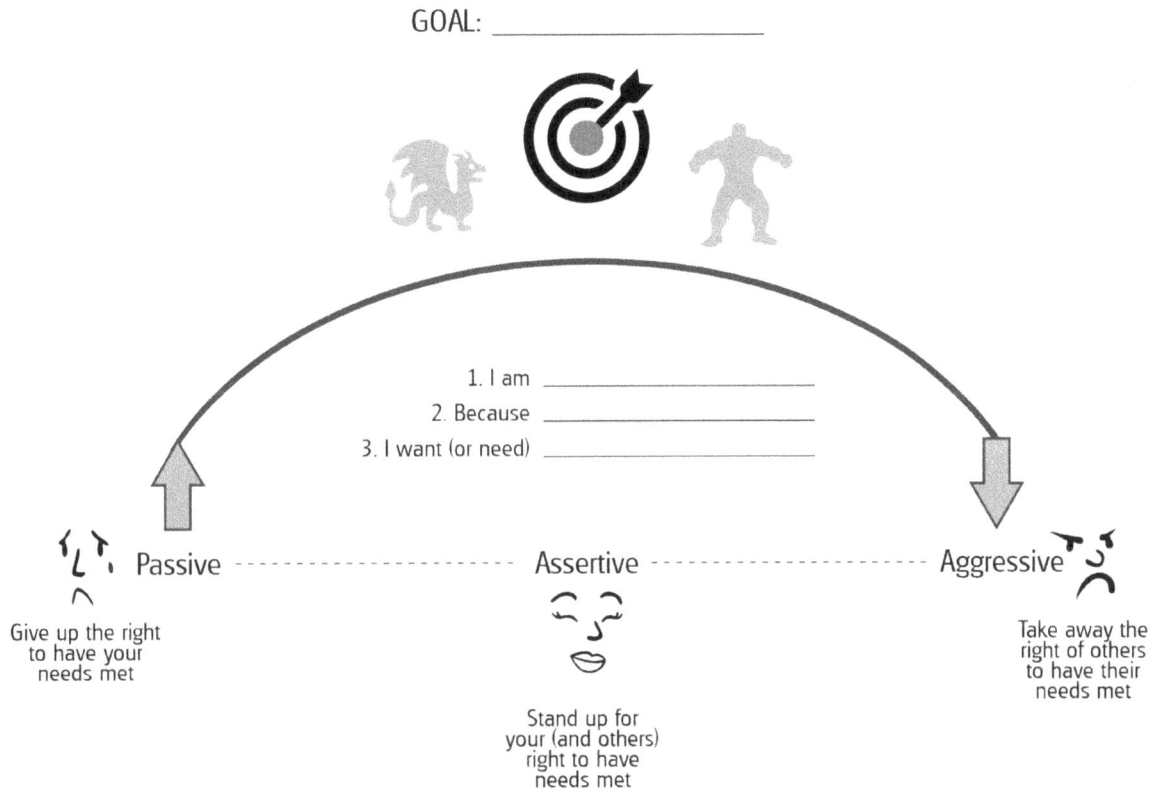

GOAL: _____

1. I am _____
2. Because _____
3. I want (or need) _____

Passive - - - - - - - - - - Assertive - - - - - - - - - - Aggressive

Give up the right
to have your
needs met

Stand up for
your (and others)
right to have
needs met

Take away the
right of others
to have their
needs met

Passive, Aggressive and Assertive: Where Do You Sit?

On the far left of the diagram is **passive.**

This means passively giving up our chance to get our needs meet. We voluntarily

like *"You choose, I'm happy with anything," "You go first, I don't mind waiting,"* or the queen of all passive phrases: *"I'm sorry,"* even though you were not at fault.

Now, while passive people tend to make great easy-going friends, the danger point is feeling **resentful**. Feelings of resentment can sneak up quickly and is not a value that anyone – particularly a passive person – usually wants to admit. This is one of the reasons why assertiveness is so important to achieve if you want to avoid feeling resentful.

Another important reason is that once your 'passive' quota has been reached, (imagine a cup that has had too much poured into it and is now leaking and overflowing) we then tend to react passive aggressively – or just plain aggressively.

On the far right of the diagram is **aggressive.**

This means taking away the rights of others to have their needs met. Let me give you an example: you are trying to enjoy your favourite nerd crush Professor Brian Cox at the Opera and someone two rows in front is having an argument on the phone – how rude! On a more serious note, aggressive communication can, and often is, intended to intimidate and take away our right to feel safe.

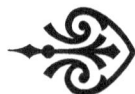

Safety Warning: If you believe that assertiveness may not be safe in your specific circumstances, such as in cases of domestic violence, or narcissistic relationships, it is crucial to seek professional advice before attempting assertive communication in case it endangers you further. *(Please see the Help Organisations section at the end of this book for more information)*

The passive communicator with their overflowing quota (or cup) will bypass the middle assertive centre and head straight on to the aggressive end. It's

and you are, because you have needs and they have been voluntarily given up all day!

Unfortunately, it is usually our loved ones (who in turn love us unconditionally) that tend to cop the brunt of this outburst. My kids like to call me the DRAGON LADY – by which they humorously help me recognise that I am needing some time out to self-nurture before returning to them more assertively (insert useless emotion of mummy guilt here). See the graphic 'dragon' on the diagram to represent this, I sometimes interchange with the 'Hulk' to explain this concept.

Common Concerns

Before I explain how easy it is to improve your assertive voice and minimise these outbursts, these are some of the common objections I routinely hear:

"Being assertive will take more time and energy."

My response: Yes, it might in the beginning, until you get more used to using (and hearing) your own assertive voice.

"I have tried, and we always seem to argue in circles."

My response: The goal is to communicate not argue. In my experience, when assertiveness is first used and doesn't work well, either the novice has accidentally begun the discussion with what the other person has done – from a motivational interviewing* perspective this is unlikely to yield desired behaviour change, or the dynamic of past arguments is a well-worn record, which we will address here in this chapter and then later in *Chapter 11 Resolve Your Conflict.*

"I would like to communicate better and be assertive, but I'm not naturally like that."

My response: You can learn to become a more confident communicator simply by using the three key sentences located in the middle of the previous picture diagram.

I am ....

Because ....

I want (or need) ....

Three Simple Sentences for Assertive Communication

Communicating assertively means standing up for your rights to have your needs met. This is done by telling people *how you feel, why you feel* that way and *what you want* to do about it. It is also useful for setting clear boundaries. Assertive communication uses these three simple sentences in this order:

The very first sentence that needs to be communicated is *how* you feel:

1. *"I am..."* (insert here how you feel, e.g., tired, disappointed, or upset etc.)

Now, this can feel very vulnerable and uncomfortable for a passive person, hence why practising on your pet is useful. Alternatively, you can also say, *"I feel..."* instead of *"I am..."* – whichever is the more comfortable for you to use. The reason why it is so important to say this first, is because it turns the other person's listening ears on.

The second sentence is *what* is making you feel that way. Be short and concise, do not waffle* on because the other person's listening ears might then turn off!

2. *"Because…………………………"* (be **specific**, be **concise** and to the **point**, e.g., your snoring has kept me awake all night, or you haven't done what you said you would, or I have had a hard day today).

Now this too can be difficult and uncomfortable because we may see microexpressions* on the other person's face. These emotions – especially pain – can make us want to take back what we are trying to say and backpedal.

This is why I encourage my clients to use other communication channels like electronic messaging, emails or even over the phone. This removes non-verbal expressions and allows us to be brave and say the three assertive sentences we need to say. This is particularly true when we are just starting out using our assertive communication. Once you are more competent at it then try more face to face.

In the third sentence, you can either use the word *need* or *want* – whichever feels better to you in the situation. In my experience, certain close relationships can use the word *need* due to its vulnerability and *want* can be used for other people and situations. However, it is your choice which one you use depending on whether *need* or *want* sounds better when you practise saying it out loud to yourself.

The third and final assertive sentence is *what* we need and it looks like this:

3. *"I need or want…"* (e.g., I need you to roll over, or I want to wear earplugs, or I want you to do what you said you would, or I need you to do what you said).

Once you've decided on your three sentences, they will sound something like this:

1. *I am* tired…
2. *Because* I have had a busy day at work, and I know we are on a budget…
3. *I want* an easy dinner tonight, what about takeaway?

Practise with yourself – who do you need to be more assertive with?

If you are already feeling **resentful**, what needs to change?

Start small and build your confidence with each use of your assertive voice.

Remember to say the sentences in this order, do not make the rookie mistake of switching up sentence one and two, and starting off with *"Because you…"* (insert red flag here)!

This rookie error usually produces an argument, so practise writing these three sentences in order and practise saying them out loud to yourself – or your dog.

NOTE: If you do use the wrong order, try again in the right order by saying, "What I meant to say was, I feel…"

Another useful way to decrease the likelihood of an argument that I recommend to my clients, is to write their GOAL at the top above the bull's eye on the previous picture diagram.

Whether the goal is to have a 'calm discussion' or to 'communicate discontent' or simply 'I want to feel heard'. This works as a reminder to stay on track and not get pulled into an argument.

We will revisit this more in *Chapter 5 Achieve Your Goals* and *Chapter 11 Resolve Your Conflict*. For now, give assertiveness a go yourself by completing these three sentences:

1. I am...
2. Because...
3. I want (or need)...

1. I am...
2. Because...
3. I want (or need)...

....

....

....

....

....

....

....

....

Also, remember the dangers of not being assertive – who wants to be resentful? Not me.

Try showing the other person the assertive three sentences and pledge to each other to only speak and reply in these three ways. If arguments persist, agree to disagree, and wait for the overnight magic.

Overnight Magic

What is this overnight magic you say? Well, after the three simple sentences have been bravely communicated and the emotions have settled, rationality can prevail.

The seed that was planted assertively the night before may yield new fruit and a better understanding the following day. You may go to bed thinking that assertive communication has not quite worked, only to wake up the next day and voilà, magic, your message was understood, and your needs are now being met.

Now, while that would be nice, having an assertive conversation does not always guarantee getting your needs met 100% of the time. What it does, is give you an opportunity to state what your needs are, so you don't spend the next three hours going over the conversation negatively in your head thinking up all the things you should have said – not to mention this style of thinking only feeds the rumination* monster.

Once you feel heard and have also listened to the other person's point of view, you can choose what you need to do to get your needs met – maybe even both of your needs met. Most of the time, simply being heard is already part of the

"Being assertive does not mean attacking or ignoring others' feelings. It means that you are willing to stand up for yourself fairly – without attacking others."

(Albert Ellis)

Summary

Communication is a dynamic process encompassing verbal and non-verbal gestures, such as smiles and frowns and even microexpressions like pain, shame, and fear. It exists on a continuum, ranging from passive (yielding your rights) to aggressive (taking away the rights of others) and sometimes, passive-aggressive.

Talking assertively means standing up for your rights by expressing your feelings, explaining why you feel that way and stating what you want to do about it. Assertiveness is being confident about what you are saying. Sometimes, it is easier to be assertive in written form and not face-to-face. For example, I often suggest to clients to text, email or even talk over the phone, rather than face to face, at least when first starting out using assertive communication.

Show the person or people you want to be assertive with, these three sentences – it is not a secret code and might help them communicate better with you. Assertiveness is sometimes easier when we are standing up for others (not just for our own rights) particularly when they do not have a voice themselves.

Remember if you do not feel safe having an assertive conversation – do not put yourself or others in danger, *(please see the Help Organisations section at the end of this book for more information).*

Three Actions to Take:

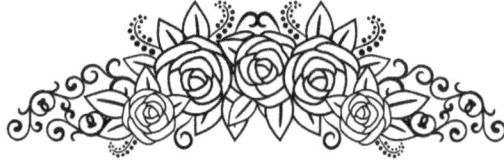

1. Examine the communication picture diagram and plot your position on the dotted line in various contexts, such as work or school, with friends, colleagues, peers, parents, spouse, children, or siblings.

Psych tip: We can change positions on this continuum in different aspects of our lives. We might be very assertive at work but wish to be more assertive at home, for example.

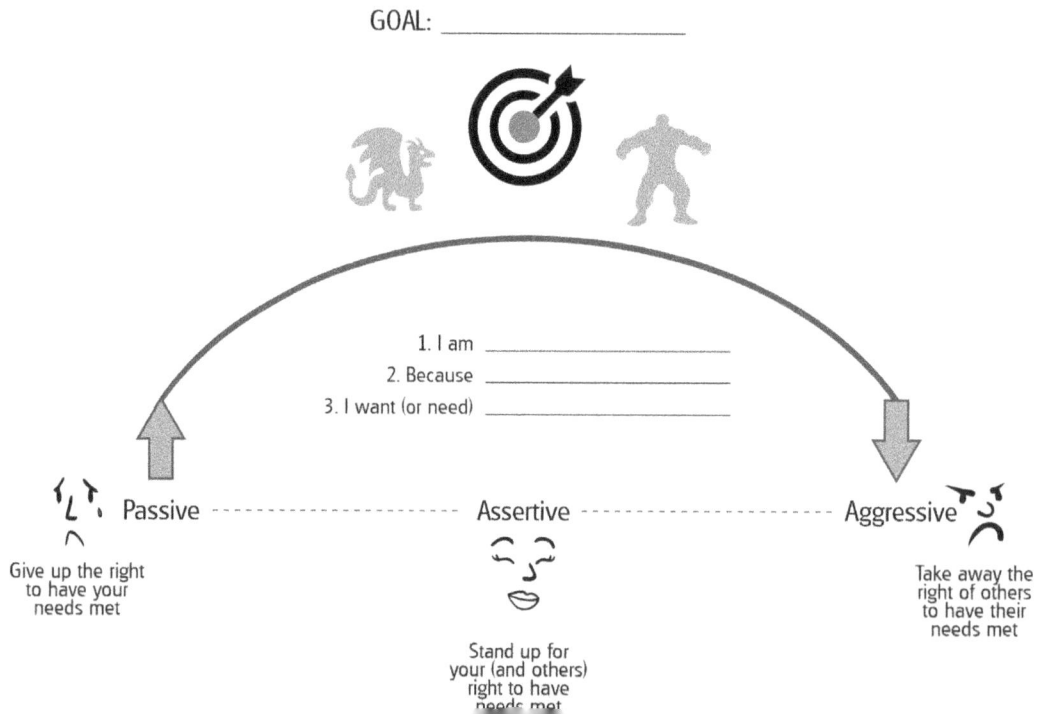

GOAL: _____

1. I am _____
2. Because _____
3. I want (or need) _____

Passive - - - - - - - - - - Assertive - - - - - - - - - - Aggressive

Give up the right to have your needs met

Stand up for your (and others) right to have needs met

Take away the right of others to have their needs met

2. Identify a small situation that you could try out your assertive communication – even minor inconveniences that you would normally grin and bear, for example, someone making an appointment when it doesn't suit you. These small irritations are opportunities to try your new assertive communication.

   For an assertive person the thought of just letting these things slide is outrageous and pointless. But for passive people, just think if all these annoyances add up, by the end of the day, your quota cup might be critically full. Each inconvenience is a chance to get your needs met. We all have different cup sizes that can also be affected by other factors, such as stress loads. So, people have different capacities: start by **noticing** your capacity as this will help you make the conscious decision to put in the effort to communicate more assertively. Who do you need to be more assertive with? Then write your goal above the bull's eye to help encourage you to stay on track.

3. Write up the three sentences in the space provided on the picture diagram. Do not just do this in your head! The action of **writing** down your thoughts and feelings can help you **understand** your mind's self-talk – a concept known as metacognition* (or thinking about thinking).

   This writing approach further prevents the formation of unhealthy habits like rumination – more on this later in *Chapter 2 Improve Your Thinking*.

   Decide which channel of communication you will use (e.g. over the telephone). Don't forget to practice saying your three sentences on safe people or pets first.

Additional Information and Resources:

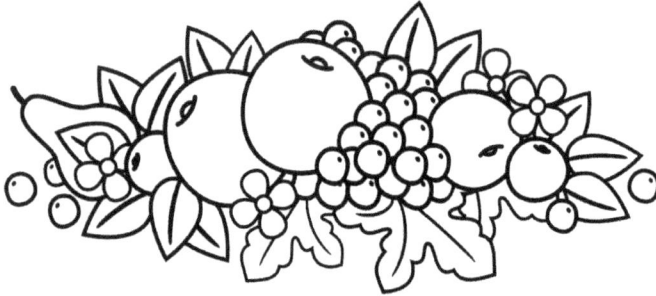

After over 15 years of practising assertiveness, I still write out what I want to say in these three sentences, I alternate between need or want, depending on which word sounds better. I practice getting it right then I usually opt for a non-face-to-face conversation and yes, I have practiced on my dog.

I still marvel when I am successful in standing up, (metaphorically), stating assertively what I want and achieving my needs. Let each win encourage your growth. Start small and build your confidence.

As we wrap up this chapter on improving your communication, let's look forward to what's to come.

Now that we've explored the significance of assertive communication and the benefits it offers, we will delve deeper into ways to enhance your thinking in the next chapter.

The pitfalls of rumination as an unhealthy thinking habit which we briefly touched on in this chapter will be explained along with other unhelpful thinking styles that are common. Keep in mind the wisdom you have gained here as it will lay the foundation for the journey ahead.

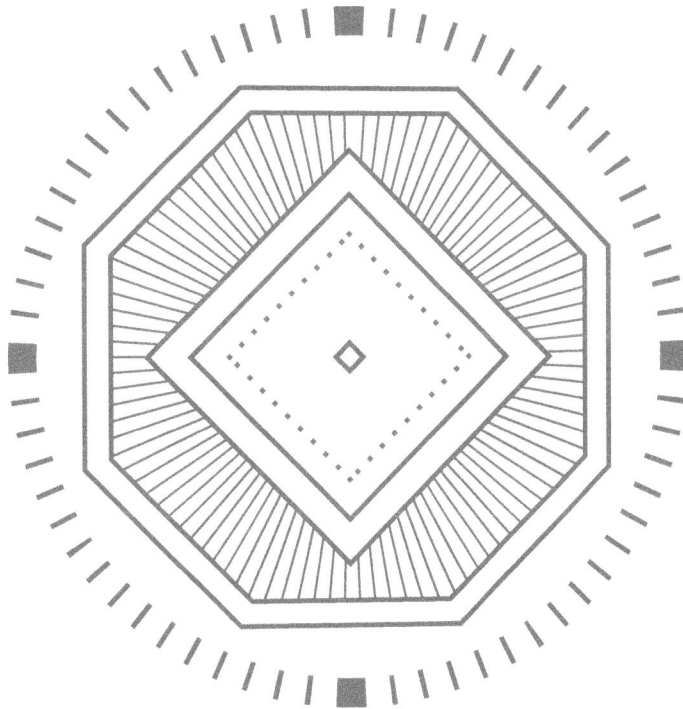

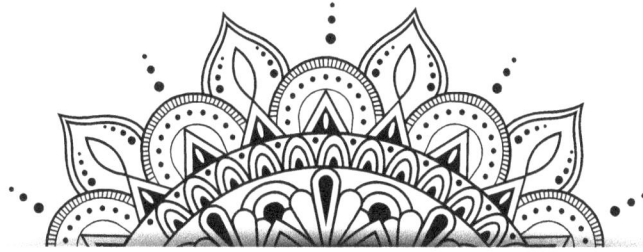

CHAPTER 2

Improve Your Thinking

"I think. Therefore, I am." (Renè Descartes)

Reality thinking is spotting and dealing with common less helpful thinking styles and is key to building a more balanced and realistic mindset.

By recognising and challenging these patterns, you can reshape how you see the world. This not only improves your mental well-being but also helps you respond more effectively to life's ups and downs, moving away from distorted views towards a clearer and more grounded perspective. Some of the benefits of challenging our unhelpful thinking habits are:

- **Improved relationships:** Realistic thinking fosters better understanding and communication in relationships. By avoiding overgeneralisations

connections based on a more accurate perception of others' intentions. Building on the last chapter's assertive communication, we will examine some of the unhelpful thinking habits that can get in the way.

- **Increased resilience:** A reality-oriented mindset cultivates resilience by encouraging adaptive responses to challenges. Instead of catastrophising or setting unrealistic expectations, individuals can approach difficulties with a balanced perspective, enhancing their ability to bounce back from setbacks.
- **Greater emotional wellbeing:** Embracing reality thinking contributes to overall emotional wellbeing. By recognising and challenging unhelpful thinking habits, individuals can experience more positive emotions, reduced mood swings and a greater sense of control over their mental state. We will uncover 7 of the most common unhelpful thinking habits and what you can do instead to combat them.
- **Enhanced problem-solving:** Reality thinking promotes a more objective and accurate assessment of situations, enabling effective problem-solving. By avoiding distorted perceptions, individuals can devise practical solutions based on realistic considerations, see *Chapter 3 Solve Your Problems*.
- **Reduced stress and anxiety:** Adopting a reality-based mindset helps alleviate unnecessary worry and anxiety. By reframing thoughts to align with facts and actual circumstances, individuals can better manage stress and maintain a calmer mental state. We will also deep dive into specifics of stress and anxiety in their own chapters: *Chapter 7 Control Your Anxiety* and *Chapter 9 Manage Your Stress*.

Negative Thoughts vs Positive Thoughts

Do we spend as much time thinking positive thoughts as we do negative ones?

According to a plethora of studies compiled over many years, we excel at negative thinking, studies found negative occurrences trigger quicker and more noticeable reactions compared to events that are positive (Carretié, Mercado, Tapia, and Hinojosa, 2001). We have a tendency to pay attention to, acquire knowledge from, and utilise negative information to a far greater extent than positive information (Vaish, Grossmann, and Woodward, 2008).

However, it is also important to note that people are diverse and their unhelpful thinking patterns can be shaped and changed through awareness and intentional efforts.

The inclination toward negative thinking varies among individuals and can be influenced by a range of factors, **nature** including personality and **nurture**, life experiences and cognitive habits. Some individuals may tend to focus more on negative aspects, while others may lean towards a more optimistic outlook.

In various situations, individuals might default to negative thinking due to stress, past experiences, or learned behaviours. Cognitive-behavioural interventions* and mindfulness* practices are examples of approaches that can help individuals recognise and modify excessively negative and unhelpful thinking patterns, promoting a more balanced and constructive mindset. We will explore some of these interventions and the 7 most common unhelpful thinking habits that present time and again in my practice.

7 Most Common Unhelpful Thinking Habits

Let's delve deeper into each of these common unhelpful thinking habits or cognitive distortions*. There are more than these 7, but to start off, have a look

1. **Personalising:** Taking on more blame than is needed for bad things, mistakenly thinking everything is your fault.
2. **Setting unrealistic expectations:** Creating super hard goals or rules that always make you feel disappointed. A tell-tale sign is wanting things to go 'perfectly' when life is messy. An example is wanting to write a book that is helpful and perfectly suited for everyone. This thinking robs us of the joy, the journey and rejoicing in the final product as it is not perfect for everyone because that goalpost is nigh impossible.
3. **Overgeneralising:** Deciding something bad will always happen based on just one small piece of evidence, drawing a conclusion about a single event, and mistakenly extending that conclusion to encompass all situations. Essentially, this involves assuming that if one event is negative, every subsequent event will also be negative. This style is linked with PTSD and other anxieties.
4. **Thinking in extremes:** Seeing things as either all good or all bad, without noticing the in-between shades of grey, like thinking life is only about constant success or failure.
5. **Catastrophising:** Making small problems seem way, way worse than they really are, like treating a tiny problem as if it is going to be a huge disaster, and it makes you super stressed, anxious, and upset.
6. **Mistaking feelings for fact:** Believing something is true just because you feel a certain way, without looking at the real facts. Referred to as emotional reasoning* as opposed to using logic. However, combining intuition with evidence, data, facts, or rational analysis can lead to more informed and well-rounded decisions.
7. **Jumping to negative conclusions:** Quickly thinking the worst will happen without enough proof, like reading a bit of a book and deciding it is going to be a sad ending without knowing the whole story. While this may be quick and efficient and provide a safety response, it can also generalise

Identifying and addressing these thinking habits is a crucial step toward cultivating a more balanced and realistic mindset. But before we do that, we also need to understand two other pertinent and often unhelpful ways of thinking.

Rumination and Automatic Thoughts*

While they share commonalities, it is important to note that rumination and automatic thoughts are distinct concepts. Rumination involves a prolonged and repetitive focus on specific thoughts, often related to negative experiences – whereas automatic thoughts are just that, more immediate, spontaneous cognitions that can contribute to rumination and emotional responses. Largely out of our awareness, these thinking styles are automatic habits. When someone consistently engages in it, it can cause emotional distress.

Rumination and automatic thoughts share a connection through the branch of cognitive processes and mental patterns:

- **Negative focus:** Both concepts often centre around negative themes. Rumination typically involves dwelling on negative experiences, while automatic thoughts can be predominantly negative and contribute to emotional distress.
- **Impact on mood:** Both rumination and automatic thoughts can significantly influence emotional states. Rumination tends to prolong and deepen negative emotions, while automatic thoughts can trigger immediate emotional reactions based on ingrained cognitive patterns.
- **Overlapping cognitive processes:** Both rumination and automatic thoughts involve repetitive and persistent cognitive processes. Rumination refers to the tendency to continuously dwell on negative thoughts, often revolving

hand, are spontaneous and rapid cognitions that arise in response to situations, often carrying emotional significance.

- **Common in Cognitive-Behavioural Therapy (CBT)*:** Both rumination and automatic thoughts are frequently addressed in cognitive-behavioural therapy (CBT), a therapeutic approach that focuses on modifying dysfunctional thought patterns. In CBT, interventions aim to identify and challenge automatic thoughts and reduce rumination to improve mental wellbeing.

Rumination has been shown to contribute to the development of anxiety and depression and worsen conditions. Rumination is a type of thinking (usually negative) going around and around in our head. Rumination is detrimental to mental health and often leads to a quicker descent into depression. It is associated with excessive negative thinking. Rumination is the repetitive and unproductive thinking that revolves around negative or distressing issues.

On numerous occasions, I have engaged in conversations about the notion that preparing for something bad to happen is considered a wise strategy. I shared this perspective until I realised the cognitive pitfall – this is a mental trap!

Rumination and worry act as snares. It might seem logical to dwell on our problems and seek a better understanding of how we ended up in a challenging situation, deciphering its meaning and anticipating potential consequences – especially when we are feeling upset.

Regrettably, much of this contemplation proves counterproductive and exacerbates our predicament. Responding to depression and anxiety by engaging in rumination and worry is akin to wielding a spade when trapped in a pit. While it might feel like delving deeper or intensifying rumination is a constructive

Should you find yourself entangled in frequent rumination or worry, consider whether there is a practical action you can currently take to address your difficulties. If there is, proceed with **taking action**, like solution-focused problem solving which we will practice next chapter.

If not, try to shift your focus to break the rumination habit by distracting yourself (try a mental task for example, like naming an animal using each letter of the alphabet).

Rumination is a habit that gets entrenched the more we do it; we will address rumination more in the next chapters. Just remember like most other habits, rumination becomes embedded the more we do it. If we wish to change the outcome, we must change our habits.

Automatic responses in our thinking are based on our belief system and is so fast it can seem automatic which is quite efficient for our brains (we will look more into these self-beliefs in *Chapter 6* on *Control Your Schema*). But for now, when something happens, we feel and think automatically because of this belief system. We need to check that our responses are rational.

Think of a time when something happened:

How did you feel? ....
What were you automatically thinking? ....
What is a more rational reasonable response? ....
I teach my young students to be a detective: ask yourself what is the evidence for and against that belief?..

The link between thoughts, feelings and behaviour is a fundamental concept in

This connection is often represented as the cognitive triangle, illustrating the interdependence of these three components:

Thoughts

Thoughts refer to the mental processes and internal dialogue that individuals have. These can be conscious or automatic, and they encompass beliefs, attitudes, interpretations, and self-talk.

Example: Thinking, *"I won't succeed in this task; I always mess things up."*

Feelings

Feelings or emotions are the subjective experiences that arise in response to thoughts or external stimuli. Emotions can range from joy and happiness to sadness, anxiety, or anger.

Example: Feeling anxious and worried due to the thought of potential failure.

Behaviour

Behaviour encompasses the actions or reactions that individuals exhibit. These actions can be influenced by thoughts and emotions and, in turn, can also affect thoughts and emotions.

Example: Avoidant behaviours towards the task or procrastinating due to the

Explanation of the Cognitive Triangle Link

Cognitive influence on emotion: Thoughts significantly influence emotions. The way individuals interpret situations or events determines how they feel about them. Different people may have different emotional responses to the same situation based on their thoughts about it. For example, being asked to chair a board meeting. Excited to be given the opportunity, or fear that you will make a highly embarrassing mistake.

Emotional influence on behaviour: Emotions play a crucial role in shaping behaviour. The way individuals feel can impact the actions they choose to take. For example, someone feeling confident may approach a task enthusiastically – while someone feeling anxious may avoid it.

Behavioural influence on thoughts and emotions: Actions can also influence thoughts and emotions. Engaging in a behaviour can either reinforce or challenge existing thoughts and feelings. For instance, successfully completing a challenging task may lead to more positive thoughts and emotions.

Practical Example:

Situation: A person is assigned a challenging work project.
Thoughts: *"I don't have the skills for this, I'm going to fail."*
Feelings: Anxiety and fear of failure.
Behaviour: Procrastination or avoidance of the task.

Understanding and modifying this connection is a key principle in Cognitive-Behavioural Therapy (CBT). Interventions in CBT often focus on identifying and challenging negative or distorted thoughts, modifying emotional responses and

Recognising and working with this link between your thoughts, feelings, and behaviour can contribute to improved mental well-being and effective coping strategies.

Challenging Our Thinking Styles and the Common Difficulties I Hear:

"What benefit would I get if I challenged my thinking?"

My response: Improving your thinking is essential to avoid jumping to incorrect conclusions and checking for faulty thinking. It helps you focus on the positive aspects of life, prevents rumination, and contributes to better mental health.

"Why is thinking more realistically, important?"

My response: Realistic thinking helps you remain balanced and resilient in the face of adversity. It is vital for your mental health and overall wellbeing.

"How can I change my thinking?"

My response: There are easy ways to combat faulty thinking patterns.

We will now examine ways to **inoculate** against the 7 common unhelpful thinking styles by practicing their **antidotes**.

Personalising means you take responsibility for everything, especially negative outcomes. Having a more balanced thinking approach by not blaming yourself for everything that goes wrong or for others' bad moods. Don't assume people act a certain way solely because of you; consider other reasons for their behaviour. For example, they may be behaving that way because they are tired, sick or had

Is personalising a style that you use?...
List other possible reasons that have nothing to do with you:

....

Setting unrealistic expectations means creating rigid standards such as unreasonable demands on self and others. Think of the phrase: *"I don't expect any more from someone than I don't expect of myself."*

You can often hear inflexible rules like, *"I must"* or *"I should"* or *"I have to."*

Consider using preferences rather than absolutes, to achieve a more balanced thinking style. For example, *"I would prefer"* as opposed to *"I must"*. Just practising this small word change can be very helpful in minimising our stress.

Is setting unrealistic expectations a style that you use?................................
Finish this sentence: I would prefer..

Overgeneralising means expecting everything to go wrong after one negative event. It can be identified by *"I will never be able to"* or labelling yourself an 'idiot'. For more balanced thinking, try to be specific rather than general in your negative thoughts and stop judging yourself and calling yourself names.

Be careful of phrases like, *"You always"* and *"I can't"* replace with, *"I cannot yet."* I often suggest treating yourself like you would treat your best friend – if you would not say it to your best friend, then why would you say it to yourself? I like to call this 'being your own best friend'.

Is overgeneralising a style that you use?...
Finish this sentence: I cannot yet..

Thinking in extremes is commonly referred to as black-and-white thinking. This is viewing situations as all or nothing, good or bad, right, or wrong, not open to any grey area in between. Try to cultivate an open-minded approach, considering possibilities rather than making definite statements. When I explain this one, especially to a younger person, I often suggest thinking about the temperature of water. It is neither boiling nor freezing as both extremes change the state of water into steam or ice. When it is ice it is inflexible, when it is steam it dissipates – try to be flexible like water, where it flows freely.

Is thinking in extremes a style that you use?...
Remind yourself that water in its state is neither extreme – get a glass of water and have a sip, is it cold or room temperature? (As you drink the water, remind yourself that there are many variations between the two extremes.)
....

Catastrophising is when we blow events out of proportion, believing that whatever can go wrong will go wrong and in a big way. Negative possibilities are often perceived as disasters, with a common thought pattern of 'what if,' contributing to anxiety. Strive for a more balanced perspective by assessing the actual likelihood of negative expectations. Practice self-reassurance, reminding yourself that there is no evidence to anticipate the worst, and consider waiting before letting worry set in. This unhelpful thinking will further be examined in *Chapter 7* which examines anxiety and its treatment in more detail.

Is catastrophising a style that you are aware of that you use?.....................................
Are you rushing to worst-case scenario? What is the likelihood of it actually happening?...

Mistaking feelings for fact or blurring feelings with reality, is when we assume that

to collect evidence to support or challenge our negative feelings. Be objective, basing conclusions on facts rather than emotions. Maintain a Daily Diary* to track your thoughts and emotions (see the daily diary example in the next section).

Is mistaking feeling for fact a style that you use?..
What are the objective facts?...

Jumping to negative conclusions, or mind reading is where we tend to draw a negative conclusion from a situation lacking enough supporting evidence or make assumptions about someone's behaviour without factual basis. Collect objective evidence, noting that only a few pieces are insufficient for a conclusive judgment. Contemplate alternative reasons that could explain someone's actions, avoiding automatically assuming the worst.

Is jumping to negative conclusions a style that you use?..
What are the facts? What are some alternative reasons?..

The initial step in addressing any of these unhelpful thinking habits is to identify and document which of the 7 unhealthy habits you observe, by using these two techniques:

Thought Monitoring Record and Daily Diary

Document your experiences using a Thought Monitoring Record*. This tool enables you to record and reflect on your thoughts, evaluating their 'helpfulness' concerning your emotions.

Thought Monitoring Record: specifically targets thoughts and emotions, aiming

For example, say the scenario is that someone isn't talking to you.

Track specific thoughts e.g. *"I did something wrong, it's my fault."*
Emotions e.g. upset and angry at self
Evidence (fact) they are not talking to me, but they are not talking to anyone else either.
Cognitive distortions e.g. personalising
Challenge negative thoughts e.g. maybe they have other stuff going on.
Balanced thought - I don't think I did anything to upset them, and I know I definitely did not intend to upset them so I will try to reach out to them tomorrow to see what is wrong.

Your automatic thoughts* are familiar because they have been your longstanding way of thinking, rooted in self-belief systems. Be open to challenge your automatic thoughts. Be a detective and gather evidence to either support or challenge them. What are the facts in the situation and seek evidence for and against your interpretation?

Consider alternative viewpoints and ask whether there is another way to perceive the situation. Evaluate how much you believe in these interpretations and whether they will help you cope or feel better.

While both a Daily Diary and a Thought Monitoring Record involve recording thoughts and feelings, they serve slightly different purposes.

Daily Diary typically involves recording a variety of information about one's day, including events, activities, and emotions. It provides a comprehensive overview of daily experiences, helping individuals identify patterns or triggers for certain emotions or behaviours. In a daily diary, you might record what you did, where

Thought Monitoring Record is more focused on tracking specific thoughts and associated emotions. It is often used in Cognitive-Behavioural Therapy (CBT) to help individuals become aware of and challenge automatic negative thoughts. In this technique, you typically write down negative thoughts as they occur, analyse them for cognitive distortions, and work on developing more balanced and realistic thoughts (see below).

Both tools can be valuable in self-reflection and therapeutic processes.

Daily Diary: record what you did, where you were, and how you felt throughout the day.

Record today's events...
Activities...
Behaviours...
Emotions..
Patterns and Triggers..

Thought Monitoring Record: specifically targets thoughts and emotions, aiming to identify and modify unhelpful thinking patterns.

Situation...
Track specific thoughts...
Emotions..
Evidence to support or not?...
Cognitive distortions..
Challenge negative thoughts..
A more balanced thought...

Thought Stopping

Instead of being on autopilot take control of your own cranial cockpit. Explore various thought control techniques, (not like in the novel *1984*, but using your own mind to keep in control) like refusing to tolerate negative thinking habits. Utilise thought-stopping*, where you interrupt negative thoughts by saying '*stop*' and imagining pleasant scenes to distract yourself. Engage in other distraction techniques*, such as keeping busy, going for a walk, singing, or practicing relaxation exercises, to prevent the escalation of less helpful thoughts.

Rehearse

Rehearse difficult situations to maintain calm and control during challenging moments. You can also use the thought monitoring record to review uncomfortable or embarrassing experiences more positively, by treating them as opportunities for growth and learning. Albeit awkward, we have all experienced them and it isn't fatal.

Worry Time

Allocate specific time, like 30 minutes each day, for negative thinking or worrying (called worry time*). Wait to respond until your thoughts are logical and defer making decisions until you are in a calmer state, more on this in coming chapters.

Rumination Story: Little Blue Wren

One morning, upon arriving at work, I opened the front door, and a little blue wren swiftly flew inside just as I was closing the door. As it flew up the hallway, it pooped all over the carpet! It continued to fly all around the office, possibly as perplexed as I, on how to aid escape.

I tried to coax it gently back into the reception area where I had opened the front door again. I held my arms out wide herding it back to freedom and then it landed on my outstretched finger! I was shocked as it sat perched looking at me and I looked at him. It was like a scene out of a *Disney* movie, apart from the singing.

There was no one else in the office and as I pondered how to get to my mobile to take a photograph, I realised I had but one chance to help it escape. I slowly walked towards the door, with the blue wren still perched upon my finger.

As I approached the open door, I heard another wren chirp in the trees just outside. Off my blue wren flew towards his friend. I have thought many times of that experience, having no photograph as proof (other than the poop I had to clean off the hall carpet) and the memory in my head. I use that experience as an analogy to explain rumination.

Rumination is a thought that goes around and around in our head. Just like the blue wren flying around and around the office. Had there been no open door to escape, I fear that the little wren would have flown around and around searching to no avail and eventually, falling from exhaustion. This is the same as our ruminating thoughts going around and around in our own head, until we are exhausted!

The open door represents a way out, an exit. And the exit for ruminating thoughts

phone. As long as some action is being taken e.g., pen writing, fingers typing, then it allows the escape of your ruminating thought from inside your head just like the escape of that little blue wren.

Rumination

Rumination involves persistently focusing on challenges and distressing thoughts, repeatedly revisiting past events, becoming preoccupied with certain thoughts, and finding it difficult to **disengage** from them. It is a **learned** strategy individuals use to grapple with their problems. Rumination is usually a time-limited process that concludes when attention shifts to other matters.

For example, if you are getting ready for work/school/exercise and you are in the shower doing the same routine day in and day out, you might find you start to ruminate over a problem, however it is time restricted because you have to get out of the shower and leave for work/school/sport.

If you are driving the same route day in and day out, you might find yourself ruminating once more. However, again it is time limited because once you arrive at your destination you become busy and do not have any **free time** to ruminate. A sign that you are ruminating is when you have thoughts like, *"Why do these things always happen to me?"* or *"What did I do to deserve this?"*

*'**Why**'* questions tend to focus on the problem, its causes, and consequences.

Rumination Diary

A rumination diary is a tool to help individuals track and manage persistent, repetitive thoughts, known as rumination. Rumination involves continuously thinking about the same thoughts or concerns without reaching a resolution. Keeping a rumination diary can be beneficial in increasing awareness of these thoughts and understanding patterns that contribute to emotional distress.

Rumination tends to occur when our minds can wander, doing repetitive tasks that do not take much concentration. For example, folding washing, or watching television that has not grabbed your attention. Identifying your **danger** times can help manage them to a minimum. The rumination diary typically includes the following components:

- **Date and time:** Record the date and time each time you notice yourself engaging in rumination.
- **Rumination trigger:** Identify the situation or event that triggered the ruminative thoughts. This could be a specific event, conversation, or even a general mood.
- **Thoughts:** Write down the specific thoughts that are circulating in your mind. Be as detailed as possible about the content of your ruminations.
- **Emotions:** Note the emotions or feelings associated with the thoughts. This helps in understanding the emotional impact of rumination.
- **Intensity:** Rate the intensity of your emotions and the strength of the ruminative thoughts on a scale, for example, from 0 - 100.
- **Cognitive distortions:** Identify any cognitive distortions present in your thoughts. Common distortions include catastrophising, and overgeneralisation.
- **Coping strategies:** Record any strategies you attempted to use to cope

- **Outcome:** Reflect on the outcome of your rumination. Did it lead to a resolution or increased distress? How did it impact your mood or behaviour afterward?
- **Alternative thoughts:** Encourage yourself to identify more balanced or alternative thoughts to challenge the ruminative ones. Consider a more realistic perspective on the situation.
- **Patterns and themes:** Look for patterns or recurring themes in your rumination. This helps in recognising triggers and developing strategies to interrupt the cycle.

Using a rumination diary provides individuals with a structured way to explore and understand their thought patterns. It can be a valuable tool in therapy for developing healthier thinking habits and implementing effective coping mechanisms to reduce the impact of rumination on emotional well-being (see below example):

Rumination Diary:
Date/time...
Trigger: What happened prior? Where were you? What were you doing?
e.g. driving to work in the car listening to news on the radio................................
Content: What were you thinking about? e.g. finances...
Feelings: How did you feel? What was the intensity 0-100 as a %?
e.g. anxious 75%, angry 20%, sad 5%...
Cognitive distortions: Were any of the distortions present?...................................
....
Coping strategies used: Were they effective or not?...
....
Consequences: How did ruminating make you feel afterwards? Better or Worse? ....
Alternative thoughts: What are more balanced or alternative thoughts?

Duration: How long did you ruminate? e.g. all the way to work 35 mins....................
Stopping: What stopped the rumination?...e.g. arriving at work............................

Once you are aware of when your **danger** times for ruminating occur and why, you can start to challenge that style of thinking by asking yourself better questions using '**how**': *"How can I solve this problem?"* or *"How can I get out of this situation?"*

Another helpful way to minimise rumination thinking is to write down your answers to the how questions. In the next chapter, we will explore how to solve problems more efficiently.

Summary

Rumination leads to poor mental health, which is why it is essential to break this pattern. This chapter also includes an explanation of 7 common unhelpful thinking styles and their countermeasures. Automatic thoughts are rapid, fleeting, and often subconscious cognitions that spontaneously arise in response to situations or events. These thoughts are immediate interpretations or judgments about what is happening, and they can be influenced by emotions, past experiences, and underlying beliefs.

Automatic thoughts play a significant role in cognitive-behavioural therapy (CBT), where individuals are encouraged to identify and evaluate these thoughts to understand their impact on emotions and behaviour. This process helps individuals recognise and challenge negative or distorted thinking patterns, leading to more balanced and constructive cognitive processes. Therefore, it is crucial to consciously shift our thinking towards more positive perspectives

Some of the helpful techniques discussed in this chapter were thought monitoring record, thought stopping, keeping a daily diary, distraction, rehearsal, and allocating worry time.

Three Actions to Take:

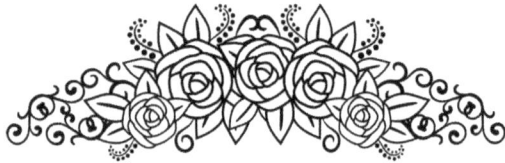

1. Identify your unhelpful thinking styles by highlighting which ones out of the 7 common unhelpful thinking styles in this chapter. Keep a daily diary for one week to help you notice which thinking styles are common for you.

List of Unhelpful Thinking Styles:

- Personalising
- Setting unrealistic expectations
- Overgeneralising
- Thinking in extremes
- Catastrophising
- Mistaking feelings for fact
- Jumping to negative conclusions

2. Keep a thought monitoring record to help you identify and challenge your unhelpful thinking styles.

3. Practice narrative therapy through journaling to explore your thoughts and feelings. Utilise the space provided to keep a rumination diary. Alternatively, if you prefer you can keep it electronically on your mobile telephone or computer.

Rumination Diary: Date/time...

Trigger: What happened prior? Where were you? What were you doing? e.g. driving to work in the car listening to news on the radio................................

Content: What were you thinking about? e.g. finances...........................

Feelings: How did you feel? What was the intensity 0-100 as a %? e.g. anxious 75%, angry 20%, sad 5%...

Cognitive distortions: Were any of the distortions present?......................
....

Coping strategies used: Were they effective or not?................................
....

Consequences: How did ruminating make you feel afterwards? Better or Worse? ....

Alternative thoughts: What is a more balanced or alternative thoughts?
....

Duration: How long did you ruminate? e.g. all the way to work 35ms....................

Stopping: What stopped the rumination?...e.g. arriving at work.............................

Daily Diary: record what you did, where you were, and how you felt throughout the day.

Record today's events...

Activities...

Behaviours..

Emotions...

Patterns and Triggers...

Thought Monitoring Record: specifically targets thoughts and emotions, aiming to identify and modify unhelpful thinking patterns.

Situation...

Track specific thoughts...

Emotions...

Evidence to support or not?...

Cognitive distortions..

Challenge negative thoughts..

More balanced thought..

....

....

....

....

....

....

Additional Information and Resources:

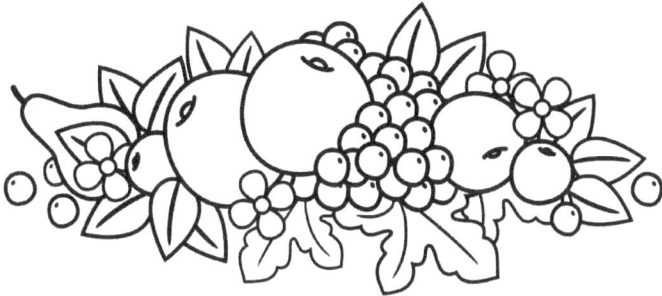

With your thinking improved and unhelpful thinking habits addressed, you are now better equipped to explore problem-solving in the next chapter which will further break the unhealthy habit of ruminating thinking.

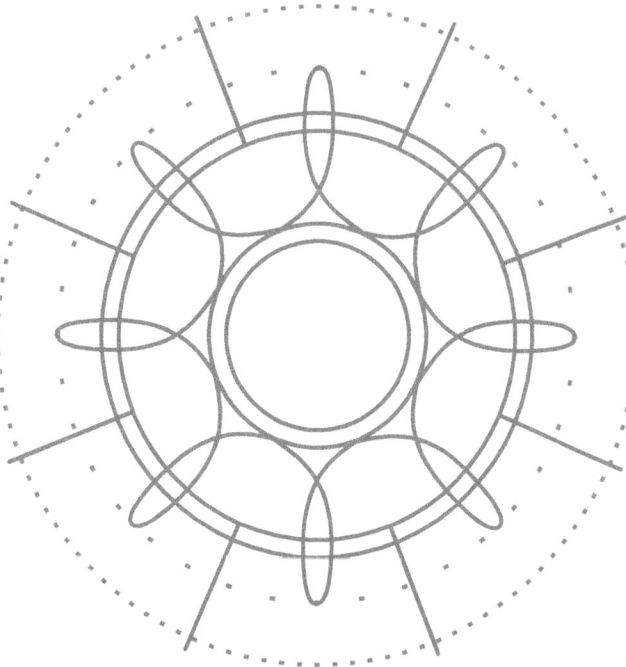

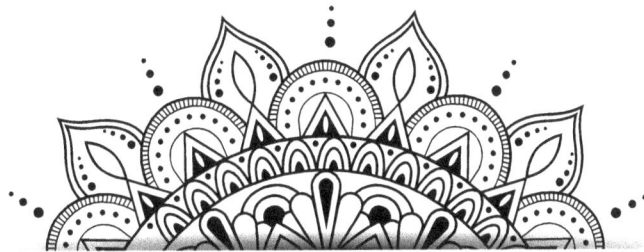

CHAPTER **3**

Solve Your Problems

"The way we see the problem is the problem." (Stephen Covey)

Problem solving is a very useful skill. This is the problem-solving method that I have used over and over throughout the years with many clients. These six steps to problem solving provide a reliable approach with a built-in alternative to overcome decision-making paralysis.

Have you ever not made a decision because you were not sure? There are several benefits to using this problem-solving method:

- six simple reliable consistent steps.
- used for a large range of problems.
- built-in alternative hack to prevent decision-making paralysis.
- helps increase your confidence in tackling problems and decision making.
- prevents or at least minimises ruminating thoughts.

Minimise ruminating thoughts and the accompanying loss of sleep just by using a pen and noting down all the options and solutions that go around in your head. Do you recall how the little blue wren story in the last chapter needed me to open the front door to escape? Your thoughts need to be able to exit your brain by an action like writing them down, this minimises habit forming rumination.

"Identify your problems but give your power and energy to solutions."
(Tony Robbins)

Common Protests to Facing Problems

Sometimes, people prefer to avoid making any decision, because it is easier to ignore the problem – until you can't anymore.

"What if I make the wrong decision?"

My response: The beauty of this failsafe approach is that you can always return to step 4, which keeps the momentum going. It is about progress and action.

"What if I like to mull things over in my head?"

My response: While you may find pondering decisions beneficial, be cautious not to fall into the trap of rumination, which is harmful to your mental health. This problem-solving method keeps you from overthinking and helps direct you towards action.

"Do I have to write it down?"

My response: While writing it down is recommended, you can also type it out on your electronic device, for example, a mobile phone. The essential thing is to perform an action (not just in your head), so it discourages ruminative thinking and helps you improve your problem-solving skills.

Problem Solving Exercise

Follow the six steps:

1. Identify what the problem is: _____

2. Write all the options

3. Evaluate each option above   Pros | Cons

4. Decide and write the best option(s)

_____

5. Action plan:

Who	What	When	Where	How

6. Did it solve my problem?
   Yes (celebrate)

   If No, go back to step 4 and choose the next best option.

Psych Tip: *Momentum-don't get stuck by not making any decision.*

How to Use this Failsafe Problem Solving Method

Step 1. Identify a problem and write it into the space provided. If it doesn't fit, consider whether it can be broken down into smaller problems as each may need a separate six steps for each problem that needs to be solved.

Step 2. Write all possible solutions/opportunities available to you. Leave lots of space for this section so you can brainstorm as many different options as possible that you can think of. Refrain from evaluating just yet as it may interrupt the flow of imagination and creativity which help you come up with as many different ideas as you can. Write down even the whacky ideas as these more fanciful choices

Step 3. Once this list is exhausted it is time to evaluate each of the options. Write the good and bad outcomes of each solution. Generally referred to as pros and cons. These positives and negatives allow you to compare each solution.

Step 4. Choose the best solution that is in front of you. Which of the pro and con appraisals highlight the best decision?

Step 5. Write the decision into an action plan. I prefer to use a table to indicate *who* will do *what when where* and *how.*

Step 6. The failsafe question. Did this solution solve your problem? If yes, celebrate and tell all your friends and use that win to give you confidence for the next problem to solve. Now if the answer is no, do not hesitate – go back to step 4 and choose the next best solution on your list.

Let's do an example together.

Step 1: Define what the problem is. Write your problem in the space provided.

A few examples to think of could be: which car/phone/formal outfit to buy, or which school/sport should your kids go to, or even, friends are coming over for dinner, so what should you cook?

Identify what the problem is: _____

Psych tip: *Ensure it is only one problem not several wrapped up together. If so, you can still use this method, but you need to do the six steps for each individual problem broken down into manageable pieces.*

Step 2: Write all the options you can think of. Be creative and think outside the box. Creative companies use organised ideation, this 'totally out there' thinking helps to generate new ideas and perspectives because it suspends the limits of conventions.

Write all the options: (one option per line)

_____

_____

_____

_____

Do not judge your options or solutions, just brainstorm as many as you can, and make sure you have enough room. Once you are used to this method, it can be entertaining to compete against yourself and come up with more – even when you think there are none.

Step 3: Now is the time to evaluate each of the options. Write a list of all the pro's and con's for each of your options. Write down all the benefits/consequences of all the good and the bad for each option.

Psych tip: I suggest working backwards, by starting with the last option and work back up the list of options. Make sure you have enough room across, maybe even use a larger piece of paper or computer once you get the hang of it.

Evaluate each option above	Pros	Cons

Step 4: Choose the best solution once you have completed all of your pro's and con's, see which option stands out the most.

Decide on the best option and write it here:

_____

Psych tip: Do not just add up all the pro's and all the con's to see which option has the most or least as some of these evaluations are weighted more important or valuable to you.

Step 5: Now is action. Create an action plan by writing:

Who, What, When, Where, How

Action plan:

Who	What	When	Where	How

Step 6: The failsafe question. Did this solution solve your problem? If yes, celebrate and tell all your friends and use that win to give you confidence for the next problem to solve.

Now if the answer is no, choose the **next best** solution on your list and continue with Action plan.

Decide and write the **NEXT** best option:

_____

Action plan:

Who	What	When	Where	How

Did this solution solve your problem? If yes, celebrate and tell all your friends and use that win to give you confidence for the next problem to solve.

Now if the answer is no, choose the **next best** solution on your list and continue with Action plan.

Continue until the problem is solved.

Summary

Problem-solving is a valuable life skill that not only addresses issues directly but also helps prevent the detrimental cycle of rumination. Rumination, characterised by repetitive and circular thinking, can contribute to poor mental health. Engaging in problem-solving provides an efficient and constructive alternative, breaking the cycle of unproductive habits and promoting mental wellbeing.

Three Actions to Take:

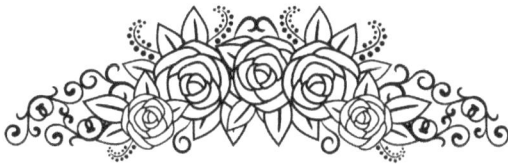

1. Practice with this problem solving six steps. Choose a small problem to start with and build your confidence.

Psych Tip: Momentum- don't get stuck by not making any decision.

Problem Solving Exercise

Follow the six steps:

1. Identify what the problem is: _____

2. Write all the options

_____

_____

_____

_____

3. Evaluate each option above   Pros | Cons

4. Decide and write the best option(s)

_____

5. Action plan:

Who	What	When	Where	How

6. Did it solve my problem?
     Yes (celebrate)

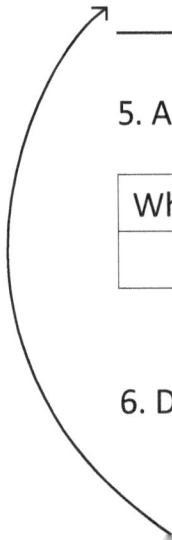

2. **Brainstorm creatively:** When listing options, be creative and aim to come up with as many solutions as possible without judgment or evaluation until you have exhausted your list of possible options.

3. Feel reassured to make a decision, knowing that the 'escape clause' at Step 6 is available. You can always revisit and revise your decision, ensuring you never get stuck in a dead-end problem-solving process or worse get stuck in decision-making paralysis.

Additional Information and Resources:

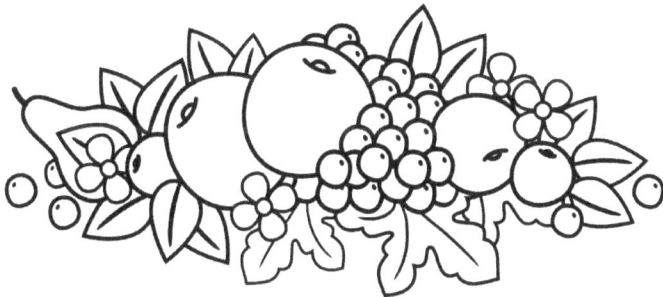

With your newfound problem-solving skills, you are better equipped to face challenges and make decisions effectively. This book will now delve into supporting individuals dealing with depression.

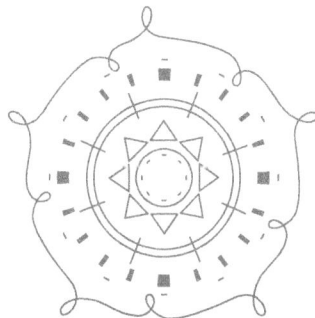

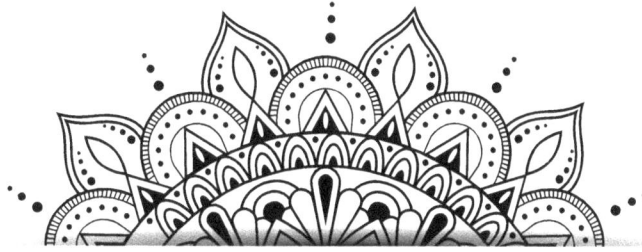

CHAPTER 4

Lift Your Depression

"It's so difficult to explain depression to someone who's never been there, because it's not just sadness." (J.K. Rowling)

Depression* can cast a large shadow over every aspect of life and drain you of all energy. This chapter offers a beacon of hope, suggesting strategies to help lift the weight of depression and regain a sense of self. Depression can feel like an endless tunnel of despair, but with the right support and strategies, it is possible to see the light at the end and regain your zest for life. Several benefits of using the strategies even just the smallest of steps are:

- Rediscover the ability to experience joy and find meaning in life.
- As depression lifts, you will find it easier to engage in healthy relationships.
- Overcoming depression can lead to increased productivity and a more satisfying life.
- Mental wellbeing is closely connected to physical health and lifting

By addressing depression, you can regain emotional strength and resilience.

The Shocking Truth

Approximately 264 million people worldwide suffer from depression, according to the World Health Organisation, making it a common but highly treatable condition.

In 2019, the *World Health Organisation* found 40 million people worldwide experienced bipolar disorder*.

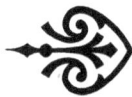

Safety Warning: If you have concerns for your safety or someone else's it is crucial to seek professional advice with a GP or closest Emergency Department.

If you suspect bipolar disorder it is recommended to seek professional advice from your GP. Bipolar disorder involves alternating depressive episodes and manic symptoms, including mood shifts, increased activity, and risky behaviour. Effective treatments, such as psychoeducation, stress reduction, and medication, exist to manage the condition and reduce the risk of suicide.

"Promise me you'll always remember: You're braver than you believe, stronger than you seem, and smarter than you think."
(A.A. Milne, Winnie the Pooh)

Learned Helplessness

Martin Seligman's proposition on learned helplessness* and its impact on depression provides an understanding into specific human behaviours that might seem unusual or counterproductive. Grasping the concept of learned helplessness opens avenues for mitigating or eliminating its adverse effects particularly in relation to depression. (Ackerman, 2018)

This behaviour is evident in animals as well. When a trainer begins working with a baby elephant, they often use a rope to tether one of the elephant's legs to a post. Despite the initial struggle, lasting for hours or even days, the elephant eventually ceases its attempts to break free and comes to accept its restricted movement. (*Wu*, 2009)

As the elephant matures and becomes physically capable of breaking the rope, it refrains from attempting to do so, having learned that resisting is futile. I sadly witnessed this in Nepal at a wildlife sanctuary.

When humans or animals believe that they lack control over their circumstances, they start to think, feel, and behave as if they are powerless.

Seligman and colleagues posited that exposing individuals to scenarios where they lack control leads to three impairments: **cognitive, motivational** and **emotional.** (Abramson et al., 1978)

The **cognitive** deficit pertains to the individual's perception that their circumstances are beyond control. The **motivational** deficit involves the individual's failure to respond to potential means of escaping an unfavourable situation.

Ultimately, the **emotional** deficit manifests as a sense of depression when the individual finds themselves in a negative situation that they believe is beyond their control.

The variety of depressive symptoms hinges on the extent and stability of **helplessness**, with the impact on self-esteem influenced by how individuals internally or externally explain their experiences.

Typical depression symptoms include changes in **emotions**, moody, irritable, empty, numb, teary, worthlessness, guilt, sad, hopeless, loss of interest and pleasure in things that were once enjoyable, tired, lack energy and motivation, worried and tense.

Typical reported changes in **cognition** (thoughts) include difficulty to concentrate, difficulty to make decisions, self-critical, self-blame, negative thoughts about self, about body image, low self-esteem, low thoughts of others, about the future and the world, thoughts about death, suicidal ideation*.

Typical changes in **behaviour** include poor attention to personal hygiene and appearance. For example, when someone arrives in slippers and hair not brushed or washed it is usually an indication they are not travelling very well (I am always amazed that they even managed to arrive for their appointment which is an extraordinary effort). Decreased peer and usual activities, self-harm, avoid family and activities, withdrawn, more alone time, easily upset and quick to anger.

Typical physical changes include low energy, changes in appetite and weight, changes in sleep patterns, difficulty sleeping or oversleeping, lowered libido, restless, agitation, aches, and pains.

Cognitive Restructuring

Cognitive restructuring* is like renovating the thought landscape of your mind. It's all about recognising those sneaky negative thoughts that can creep in and mess up your mental decor. I guess it's a bit like weeding a garden – the trick is to spot the pesky thoughts before they take over.

In a previous chapter, we examined improving your thinking to avoid jumping to incorrect conclusions and checking for faulty thinking. It helps you focus on the positive aspects of life, prevents rumination, and contributes to better mental health.

Cognitive behavioural therapy* (CBT), and other therapies are like the architects and interior designers of your mental space, helping you tear down the walls of negativity and build a more positive foundation. It is fascinating how thoughts, feelings and behaviours are all interconnected. Change one and it can have a ripple effect on the others.

But, you know, catching those cognitive distortions is no easy feat. It's like trying to catch a sly fox – they're quick, and by the time you notice them, they've already done their damage. So, it's like mental ninja training – learning to be aware and quick on your mental feet.

Common protestations I hear when treating depression:

"I can't overcome depression; it's too overwhelming."

My response: While depression can be incredibly challenging, it is treatable, and many have successfully navigated their way out of it. With the right support and

"Seeking help for depression is a sign of weakness."

My response: Seeking help is a courageous step toward healing, and it does not indicate weakness, it is a brave sign of inner strength. It shows self-awareness and a commitment to improving your mental health.

"I've tried various treatments for depression, and nothing works."

My response: Depression treatments can be highly individual. What didn't work before may not be the right approach for you. This chapter explores different strategies to help you find what works best for you.

Rumination and Disrupted Routines

I became more aware of this phenomenon when I noticed patients' depression seemed to get worse when they were off work on sick leave due to an injury. With the normal routine disrupted, rumination if it was slightly present before, was able to ramp up with all the extra time the patient had to recuperate. Covid was another time I experienced this decline in mental health. I gave several online presentations addressing rumination and devising new routines that included:

Self-monitoring records, behavioural activation*, activity menus, activity scheduling, thought records, and thought challenging.

These are cognitive behavioural therapy (CBT) techniques that help individuals identify and change negative thought patterns and behaviours that contribute to depression.

Psychoeducation

Psychoeducation* is learning more and gaining a thorough understanding of mental health like depression, its effects, management, and treatment options.

Emotional Literacy

Emotional literacy refers to the ability to recognise, understand, express, and manage one's own emotions, as well as the capacity to comprehend and respond effectively to the emotions of others. It involves being aware of and having a nuanced understanding of various emotions and being skilled in navigating and expressing these feelings in a socially appropriate manner.

Emotional literacy is essential for building healthy relationships, effective communication, and overall wellbeing. I have a fun game called *Emotional Bingo* that children enjoy playing whilst they develop a wider emotional vocabulary.

Daily Mood Monitoring Chart

Utilise the daily chart: https://www.blackdoginstitute.org.au/wp-content/uploads/2020/04/19-dailymoodchart.pdf to provide an overall assessment of your mood on a day-to-day basis (Rate from 1 to 10, where 1 is the worst and 10 is the best).

It is helpful to take this chart with you to your appointment with your GP or healthcare professional, especially if you are concerned about your concentration ability, or dealing with memory issues, which are common with depression.

Medications

Record all current and past medications, including what you took, when, for how long, and the effects (both positive and negative), along with reasons for discontinuation. Bring this list with you when you see your GP.

Self-Monitoring Record

Used to track and analyse thoughts, moods, and behaviours associated with depression. They enhance awareness, identify negative thought patterns, track daily activities, set goals, and provide feedback for therapy. These records aid in understanding and managing depressive symptoms while allowing active participation in treatment.

Situation that triggered low mood? Who were you with? Where? When?
....
Thoughts? (or images /memory) ....
Emotions & body feelings? Rank strength of each as a %..
Response: What did you do? How did you cope?...

Elevating Your Activity Level

A strategy to counter depression involves a simple increase in your activity level, particularly in enjoyable activities – those that bring joy – and addressing your list of tasks and responsibilities. It is crucial to approach this realistically and in an achievable manner, setting yourself up for success. Elevating your activity level offers several benefits:

Activity contributes to an improved mood. Engaging in some form of activity redirects your mind, providing a different focus. Even small steps can instil a sense of moving forward, regaining control of your life, and achieving something – a feeling of accomplishment. You might even discover pleasure and enjoyment in the activities you undertake.

Activity alleviates fatigue. Unlike the conventional need for rest when physically tired, depression calls for a different approach. Increased sleep and sedentary behaviour can exacerbate lethargy and fatigue. Being active prevents your mind from dwelling on depressive thoughts, averting an escalation of negative feelings.

Activity enhances mental clarity. Once you initiate activity, you may find yourself gaining a different perspective on life's challenges. The shift in focus brought about by engaging in activities can lead to clearer thoughts.

This approach, utilising behavioural strategies such as participating in enjoyable activities and addressing small tasks, serves as a method to break the cycle of depression and promote positive change.

Enjoyable Activities Menu

Have a look at these examples and add your own in the space provided, write all the things you enjoy doing, or used to enjoy doing (you can ask a trusted friend or family member to help you remember) e.g. riding your bike, walking your dog, reading a book, or taking a bath.

- Watch your favourite TV show, watch a comedy, go to the movies.
- Try a new food, or a new place to walk, try new music.

- Self-care – go for a massage.
- Cook yourself a favourite meal, or go out for food.
- Create, paint, draw, doodle.
- Shop, read all the comical cards in the store.
- Nature- go for a walk in the garden, plant something, buy some flowers.
- Pet an animal, volunteer at the animal shelter.

....

....

Behavioural Activation

Behavioural activation is a method employed particularly in the initial phases of treating depression. Individuals experiencing depression may struggle with the motivation and energy to accomplish fundamental, health-promoting daily activities.

This struggle can lead to isolation and compromised well-being, exacerbating the depression and creating a detrimental cycle of diminishing motivation and worsening depressive symptoms.

Use some of the enjoyable menu items to plan a weekly activity schedule. These activities should be straightforward, like completing household chores, taking a stroll, or speaking to a friend. Although these tasks may appear mundane, they can be challenging for someone grappling with depression. Having someone else to help collaboratively craft a plan with you- like a friend, family member, GP, or therapist, can help determine when tasks can be undertaken and address any potential obstacles in advance.

Weekly Activity Scheduling

	MON	TUE	WED	THU	FRI	SAT	SUN
Morning							
Afternoon							
Evening							

Easy Thought Record

Situation: Who? What? When? Where?...
....

Feeling: How did you feel? How strongly between 0-100?.. %

Thoughts: What was going through you mind? Any images or memories?....................
....

Thought Monitoring Record

In *Chapter 2*, we used this technique, and it is also pertinent here for managing depression. It helps us pinpoint negative automatic thoughts, recognise connections between events and cognitions and comprehend the interconnections between thoughts, emotions, and bodily sensations – as well as questioning and

Thought Monitoring Record: specifically targets thoughts and emotions, aiming to identify and modify unhelpful thinking patterns.

Situation...

Track specific thoughts...

Emotions...

Evidence to support or not?...

Cognitive distortions..

Challenge negative thoughts...

More balanced thought..

How Journaling Aids in Managing Depression

In the space provided practice using this book as a journal, this is beneficial in several key ways when coping with depression.

- **Enhances self-awareness:** journaling serves as a tool to deepen your understanding of yourself. Expressing your thoughts and emotions in writing brings them to the surface.
- **Facilitates expression:** writing in a journal allows you to articulate your thoughts and feelings. This process can reveal previously unrecognised issues or sources of distress. You have the option to keep your journal private or share it with your therapist, who can assist in identifying important aspects and using them to support your progress.
- **Empowers personal control:** amid the swirl of thoughts and worries, putting pen to paper can bring a sense of order and control, when we write things down, they can feel more manageable.

How Journaling Supports Your Treatment for Depression

Journaling empowers you to play an active role in your treatment, providing a constructive way to contribute to your wellbeing. It aids in recognising when you need additional support and allows for a shift in your perspective through positive self-talk.

Benefits of Journaling:

- **Empowerment and self-help:** by maintaining a journal, you take proactive steps to improve your wellbeing, fostering a sense of empowerment. It becomes a tool to identify when extra support is required.
- **Shift in perspective:** journaling offers the opportunity for positive self-talk, allowing you to alter your viewpoint and cultivate a more optimistic mindset.
- **Pattern recognition:** keeping a journal helps you track symptoms, enabling the identification of potential triggers for depression. Recognising patterns, such as worsening symptoms during specific times, under stress, or in challenging relationships, empowers you to be aware of triggers in the future.
- **Insight over time:** regularly reviewing older entries provides insight into your progress over time. By noting trends, you can gauge whether you are feeling better, worse, or the same. This retrospective analysis serves as a red flag for seeking additional help or a reassurance of your progress.

Journaling Tips:

- **Free expression:** allow your thoughts to flow freely and write about anything that comes to mind.
- **Consistency is key:** aim to journal regularly, ideally every day, for around 10-20 minutes. Find a quiet and relaxed time and place, such as before bedtime, to minimise distractions.
- **Experiment with different approaches:** explore various journaling techniques, such as writing letters to yourself or to loved ones who are no longer present. You can even compose comforting words to yourself based on what you believe your loved ones might say.
- **Maintain a balanced tone:** while expressing your thoughts, try to avoid a consistently negative tone. If you find your writing becoming overly negative, make an effort to shift your focus to more positive aspects.

....
....
....
....
....
....
....
....

Ways to Lift Your Depression

Choose one of the techniques listed to try such as psychoeducation, emotional literacy, or journaling.

Thoughts and self-monitoring: try to identify and challenge negative thought patterns that contribute to depression. Use the self-monitoring record and daily mood monitoring chart to gain insight into your emotional patterns and challenge negative thoughts and develop a healthier mindset.

Behavioural activation: engage in activities that bring you a sense of accomplishment and pleasure. Create an activity menu, keep a weekly activity schedule, and plan your activities to foster positive experiences.

Summary

This chapter offers strategies to alleviate depression, emphasising the potential for recovery with the right support. It explores the prevalence of depression globally, encourages seeking professional help and introduces the concept of learned helplessness.

Cognitive Behavioural Therapy (CBT) techniques, such as cognitive restructuring, psychoeducation, and emotional literacy, are highlighted. Tools like the Daily Mood Chart and journaling are recommended for self-awareness and expression. The importance of elevating activity levels through behavioural activation is emphasised, with practical tools provided.

Three Actions to Take:

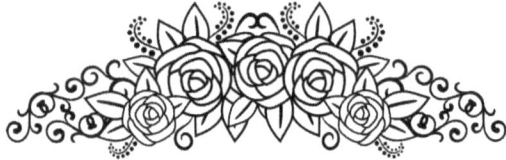

Begin monitoring your thoughts and mood daily, and challenge negative thought patterns.

Develop a plan for behavioural activation, creating your own activities menu and keep an activity schedule.

Explore CBT techniques such as thought monitoring records to help challenge thoughts, to address your depression.

Additional Information and Resources:

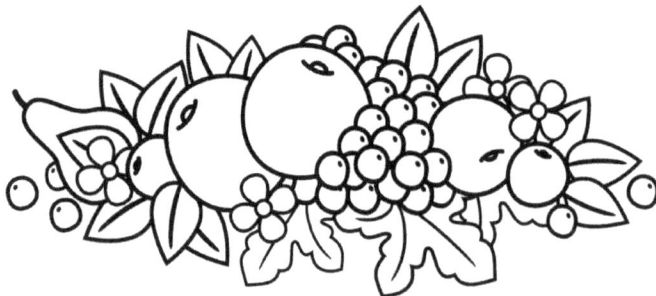

In the following chapter, we will delve deeper into additional strategies and resources to help you lift your depression, and the importance of seeking professional help when needed. Remember that you do not have to face depression alone and help is available, (*please see the Help Organisations section*

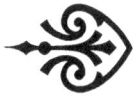

Safety Warning: *Depression can be dangerous, so it is very important to take it seriously. Please make an appointment to speak to your doctor about supports available. In case of suicidal thoughts, please reach out to LIFELINE at 13 11 14, available 24/7 to provide help and support or attend your nearest Emergency Department.*

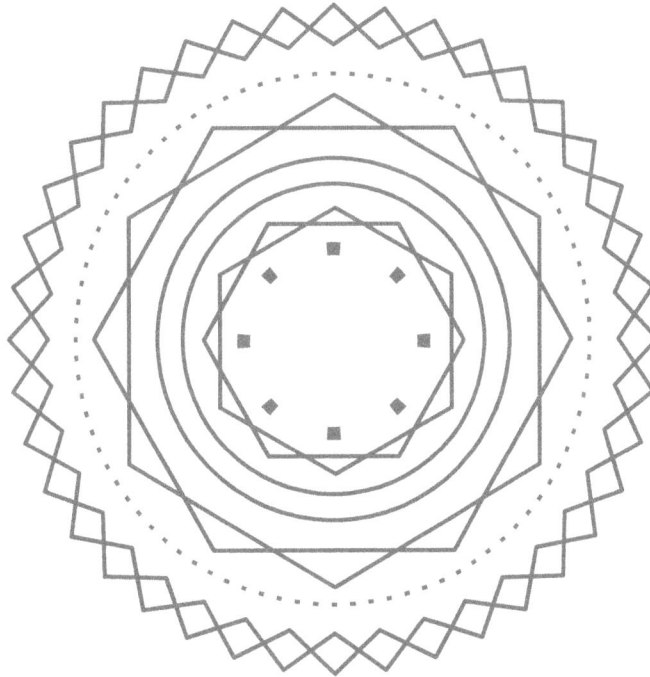

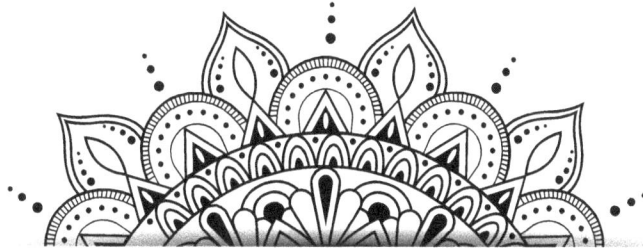

CHAPTER 5

Achieve Your Goals

"Those who have a 'why' to live, can bear with almost any 'how'."
(Friedrich Nietzsche)

Goal setting is the process of identifying specific, measurable, achievable, relevant, and time-bound objectives that an individual aims to accomplish, providing a clear roadmap for progress and success. The quote above stresses the importance of purpose, and we will explore this and Seligman's positive psychology findings in this chapter. Goal setting is not just a mundane task, but a profound practice.

In the following sections, we will delve into the five key benefits that make goal setting a pivotal tool in your life's toolkit:

- A sense of purpose: we will explore how setting goals can infuse your life with meaning and direction.

- Achieving what you truly desire: unravelling the idea that goals can help you attain your aspirations, not someone else's expectations.

- The power of SMART goals: an in-depth examination of the SMART criteria (Specific, Measurable, Achievable, Relevant, Time-bound) to supercharge your goal setting.

- Mastering time management and results: how goal setting can revolutionise your life by improving time management and seeking professional guidance through personal or business coaching.

- Action, planning, and purpose: the trio that drives goal setting and help convert dreams into reality.

Studies

Studies in the Journal of Consulting and Clinical Psychology by Epton, Currie, and Armitage (2017) have shown that goal setting has a statistically significant effect on behaviour. To examine the positive effect of goal setting on individual behaviour, this study tells us that goal setting can motivate us to adjust our behaviours in accordance with the accomplishment of our aspirations.

If you are a procrastinator, you will likely change your ways once you begin plotting your success through goal setting.

People who write down their goals are significantly more successful in accomplishing them than those who did not. In a 2007 study conducted by fellow psychologist Prof. Gail Matthews, it was revealed that those who commit their goal setting in

of what they wanted to accomplish in life. It confirms that setting goals in writing makes them tangible and realistic.

"People are not lazy. They simply have impotent goals—that is, goals that do not inspire them." (Tony Robbins)

SMART goals are a mnemonic acronym that represents a framework for creating effective and well-defined goals. The acronym SMART stands for:

- **Specific:** clearly define the goal, avoiding ambiguity. Specify what you want to achieve, why it's important, and how you plan to accomplish it.
- **Measurable:** establish criteria for measuring progress and determining when the goal is achieved. This provides clarity on what success looks like and helps track your advancement.
- **Achievable:** ensure that the goal is realistic and attainable. It should be challenging enough to motivate you but feasible with the resources and time available.
- **Relevant:** the goal should align with your broader objectives and be relevant to your overall mission or purpose. It should contribute meaningfully to your long-term aspirations.
- **Time-bound:** set a specific timeframe for achieving the goal. This creates a sense of urgency and helps prevent procrastination. It also allows you to monitor progress effectively.

Using the SMART criteria helps individuals create goals that are clear, measurable, and actionable, increasing the likelihood of successful implementation and accomplishment. Be sure to have someone to keep you accountable (my son calls himself my shopping sponsor to keep me accountable to not over shop).

Personal Development Coaching

Create a mind map: list all the areas important in your life (these are just examples you can add your own or change these).

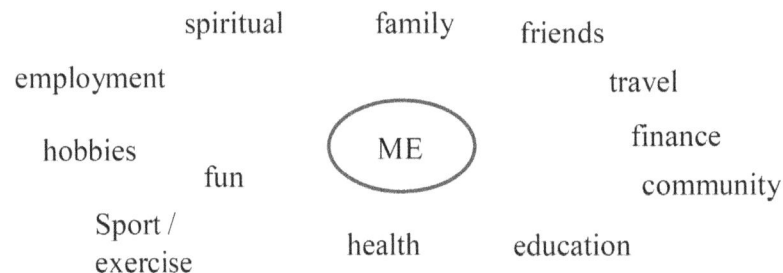

spiritual   family   friends

employment   travel

hobbies   (ME)   finance

fun   community

Sport / exercise   health   education

SMART goals

Choose one of these areas that you want to work on achieving your SMART goal:

My area is ………………………………….e.g. travel……………………………………………………….

When writing your SMART goal, make sure it is Specific, Measurable, Achievable and Relative to the area chosen above, Time-bound, and positive.

Example: My SMART goal is I am spending $1,000 on my overseas holiday in January.

Psych Tip: *Try to write goal as a positive and not negative. For example, positive goal – I am wearing my favourite size 12 blue dress on my birthday. Instead of negative goal – I want to lose weight.*

Sometimes your goal sentence may need tweaking to truly inspire and motivate you. Use these measures to help you write the goal sentence: (who), (how),

For example, (who) I am (how) spending (what) $1,000 (where) overseas holiday (when) January.

Strategies

Now, we need to write the strategies for the goal. Strategies are the major steps you need to take to achieve your goal on time.

Psych tip: *it is easier to begin with the achieved goal and work backwards, see the examples below:*

Strategy 5: I am spending $1,000 on my overseas holiday in January.
Strategy 4: Start saving.
Strategy 3: Choose the best option.
Strategy 2: Ways to increase $$$.
Strategy 1: How much $ do I have now?

Actions

Actions are the daily to-do list for each strategy.
For example: Strategy 1 – *How much $ do I have now?*

Actions:
- *Check my bank account balance*
- *Count $ in wallet or savings tin*
- *List all bills due to pay out*
- *List all income due to come in*

Strategy 2 – *Ways to increase $$$*

Actions:
- *Brainstorm all the ways*
- *Draw up a budget*
- *Only withdraw once a month*
- *Delete online shopping /betting apps*

Your turn at goal setting

Choose one of the areas from your mind map that you want to achieve in:

My area is ....

My SMART goal is ....

My Strategies are ....

....

....

....

Psych Tip: I recommend building in rewards along the way and incorporate into the last strategy as a celebration of what your goal is.

My Actions for each Strategy are:

....

....

....

....

Psych tip: *If you hit an obstacle when conducting your actions, ask yourself why? Is it something you find hard? Is there an alternative way to action it? How can you achieve it next week? If possible, have a discussion with a trusted friend, sponsor, or life coach. Remember you can also use your problem solving from Chapter 3 here as well.*

Readiness to Change*

The readiness to change graph is a visual representation that assesses an individual's willingness and preparedness to make a specific change in their behaviour, habits, or life circumstances. This graph typically involves plotting two key factors:

Importance of Change **(Y-axis):** This measures how significant the change is to the individual. It is often rated on a scale from 0 to 10, with 0 indicating low importance and 10 indicating high importance. Individuals consider why the change is necessary and how much it matters to them.

Confidence in Change **(X-axis):** This measures the individual's confidence in their ability to make the desired change successfully. Like the importance of change, it is usually rated on a scale from 0 to 10, with 0 indicating low confidence and 10 indicating high confidence. This aspect reflects the individual's belief in their capacity to overcome challenges and obstacles.

By plotting these two factors on a graph, you can visually see where you stand in terms of readiness to change. The resulting position on the graph provides insights into your psychological state regarding the contemplated change. Different quadrants of the graph may indicate various stages of readiness:

- **High Importance, High Confidence:** individuals in this quadrant are typically ready and motivated to make the change. They understand the importance of the change and believe in their ability to succeed.
- **High Importance, Low Confidence:** people in this quadrant may recognise the significance of the change but lack confidence in their ability to achieve it. They may benefit from additional support or strategies to boost their confidence, see the bonus offer 3 section for coaching resources towards the end of this book.
- **Low Importance, High Confidence:** Individuals here might be confident in their abilities, but they may not see the change as particularly important. This situation may require reassessment of priorities or goals. Motivational interviewing may be beneficial.
- **Low Importance, Low Confidence:** This quadrant indicates low readiness for change, with both the importance and confidence factors being low. In such cases, individuals may need to re-evaluate the necessity and potential benefits of the proposed change. Motivational interviewing may be beneficial, see the bonus offer 3 section for coaching resources towards the end of this book.

Understanding one's readiness to change can be a valuable tool in goal setting, behaviour modification, or any process that involves personal development. It helps individuals tailor strategies and interventions based on their current psychological state and increases the likelihood of successful and sustainable change.

Importance
to you to
make the change

Readiness to change

Confidence that you
will be able to change

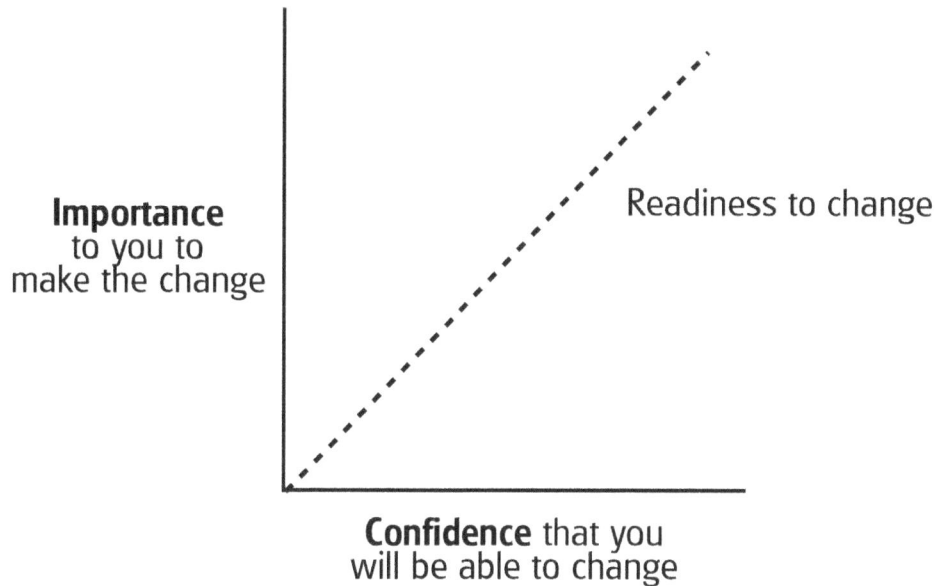

Several factors can influence an individual's readiness to change. Understanding and addressing these factors can contribute to enhancing readiness and increasing the likelihood of successful behaviour change. Here are some key factors:

- **Awareness and understanding:** having a clear understanding of the benefits and reasons behind the desired change can increase motivation. Awareness in recognising the current state and potential consequences of existing behaviours.
- **Readiness to learn:** openness to information by being receptive to new information and perspectives. Educational resources that provide guidance and information about change. Like this Challenge Journal book!
- **Stages of change*:** readiness assessment in understanding which stage of change an individual is in (pre-contemplation, contemplation, preparation, action, maintenance) helps tailor interventions.

- **Goal clarity:** specific goals clearly defining the desired outcome and breaking it into manageable steps. SMART goals are Specific, Measurable, Achievable, Relevant and Time (bound).
- **Cognitive dissonance*:** recognising discrepancies and acknowledging inconsistencies between current behaviour and desired goals can motivate change. Using the daily diary and thought monitoring record from *Chapter 2* to challenge unhelpful thinking.
- **Coping skills:** stress management by developing effective coping mechanisms for stress and setbacks. This will be explored in *Chapter 9* Manage your Stress. Problem solving skills shown in *Chapter 3* enhances the ability to overcome obstacles.

Understanding these factors and tailoring interventions to address individual needs can significantly contribute to increasing readiness to change and fostering successful behaviour change.

Eisenhower Matrix as a Time Management Tool

Have you ever wondered where all the time goes?

We all have the same amount of time, 24 hours in our day, but some people seem to achieve a lot more in that same amount of time. Have you ever wondered if there is something others know that you don't?

The Eisenhower Matrix, or Urgent-Important Matrix, is a time management tool that helps individuals prioritise tasks based on their urgency and importance. The matrix categorises tasks into four quadrants, each representing a different level of **urgency** and **importance**:

IMPORTANT

URGENT

DO IT!
Crisis
Sick
Emergency
Bill (Telstra $$)

DO IT (when)
Passion
Dreams
Goals

DELEGATE IT
Things other people
want you to do

DUMP IT
Mindless scrolling
Eg. FB & Binge
watching TV,
ruminating!

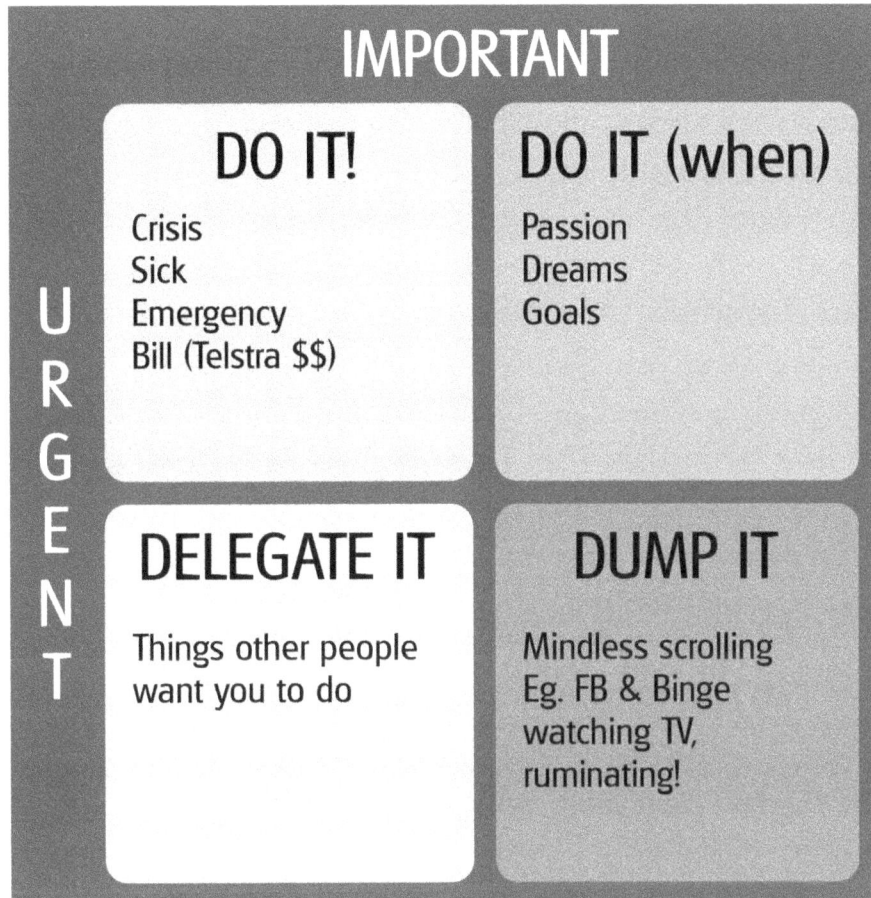

Urgent and Important (Quadrant I Do it!):

- Tasks in this quadrant are both urgent and important. They require immediate attention and should be dealt with as a top priority. Examples include crises, deadlines and bills due, for example.

Important, but Not Urgent (Quadrant II Do it (when)):

- Tasks in this quadrant are important for long term goals but not necessarily

becoming urgent later or worse, forgotten! Examples include strategic planning, relationship building, and skill development. The passion and dreams that juice your mojo belong here, the vision that gives you a sense of joy and fulfillment. The projects you do that you lose time because you are in mental flow* like writing a book perhaps.

Urgent, but Not Important (Quadrant III Delegate it):

- Tasks in this quadrant are urgent but may not contribute significantly to your long term goals. They often involve distractions and interruptions that should be minimised. Examples include some emails, meetings and certain phone calls. Urgent tasks that other people want you to do goes in this quadrant and pulls your time away from the other quadrants.

Not Urgent and Not Important (Quadrant IV Dump it):

- Tasks in this quadrant are neither urgent nor important. They are typically time-wasting activities that should be minimised or eliminated. Examples include excessive social media use, some routine tasks, and trivial activities.

The key idea behind the Eisenhower Matrix is to help individuals focus on tasks that align with their long-term goals and priorities. By visually organising tasks into these four quadrants, individuals can make more informed decisions about how to allocate their time and energy.

Here is a simple approach to using the Eisenhower Matrix:

Identify tasks: List all the tasks you need to accomplish.
Categorise tasks: Write each task in the appropriate quadrant based on its

Prioritise quadrants: Attend to tasks in Quadrant I first, followed by Quadrant II. Be careful to monitor and minimise time spent on tasks in Quadrants III and IV.

Owning your own business seems to affect the time you have available – because you don't have any! It is easy to stop doing your passion projects because there are so many other urgent competing roles and requests. **Important** tasks cover the two columns across the top, **Urgent** tasks go on the left side of the two rows. So, you end up with four quadrants – which I call 'Do it (now)', 'Do it ...(when)', 'Delegate to do it' and 'Don't do it too much or Dump it'.

What can often happen if you are not aware and organised, the Urgent Important crises are relentless and very stressful – it is better to plan the deadlines ahead of time if possible in the Important, but not Urgent quadrant. This is the top right quadrant called 'Do it...(when)' so put a date to complete it by. This way you can prevent it from becoming a stressful Urgent and Important crisis or overdue/expired.

You will still most likely have the occasional emergency or crisis in the Urgent Important quadrant but not as many, so you do not have to be under constant stress (which we will look more at Stress Management in *Chapter 9*). The other two quadrants can extract a lot of your precious time like big black holes. The Urgent but not Important quadrant can be the largest drain on your time. It often involves distractions and interruptions that could be minimised.

Examples include some emails, meetings, and certain phone calls. Urgent tasks that other people want you to do particularly because they have left it until the last minute and their stress becomes your stress!

This is when the passive helpful person starts to get resentful – remember *Chapter*

away from the other quadrants – like your long-term dreams and passion! I have two psych tips for this perilous situation.

Psych tip #1: *Ask yourself if you could **hire** a skill rather than you spending time doing it especially if you do not enjoy doing it. For example, ironing, cleaning, chopping wood, designing a website, bookkeeping, or documenting system processes.*

Psych tip #2: *If someone asks, "Have you got a minute?" which is code for an hour, you can politely say, "No, I would like to help you however I am doing this at the moment, I am free (check diary for an available spot) at this time/date." Remember your assertiveness!*

The last quadrant is Not Urgent and Not Important. This is time wasted with endless scrolling on social media for example. While some down time is important, it is imperative that if you want more time for the **Important** quadrants, you have self-restraint here.

Has anyone lost almost two hours on Facebook before you realise? Asking for a friend, of course.

Another important point is that unhelpful ruminating thinking also belongs here and steals time away from the other quadrants. Time saved here from not ruminating could be time spent in another quadrant like your important but not urgent passion and enjoyment goals.

Regularly reviewing and updating the matrix helps you adapt to changing priorities and ensures that you stay focused on tasks that contribute most to your overall happiness and goals. It is a practical tool for improving time management and

How Goal Setting Helped my Journey

Becoming a registered psychologist requires a minimum of six years of study, most of which is at university, followed by an internship upon graduation.

After that and during the period awaiting registration, I trained to be a business and life coach. My aspiration was to work as a psychologist in schools, but conventional knowledge at that time (over 20 years ago) mandated a teaching degree prior to psychology degree.

Upon completing the personal development coaching course, I enlisted a life coach to support and motivate me as I worked towards my goals. Armed with a readiness for change and a cultivated sense of learned optimism, I applied for a position as a psychologist in schools.

Successfully securing the position, I became part of a new small group of psychology recruits tasked with working in schools as a school counsellor and simultaneously studying a teaching degree. Over the dedicated 18-month period, I found great satisfaction in the endeavour, with a yearning for more, I extended my studies for an additional year, earning a Master's in Education with a focus on Emotional Disturbance and Behavioural Disorders (EDBD).

I share this story to underscore the significance of having clear SMART goals, without which I don't think I could have achieved it. The photograph on the cover of this book celebrates a competitive gym goal victory and the first prize was a photo shoot.

"You never fail until you stop trying." (Albert Einstein)

Summary

This chapter focused on the topic of achieving goals. The chapter cites studies showing the significant impact of goal setting on behaviour, emphasising that individuals who write down their goals are more likely to succeed. A practical approach is provided, encouraging readers to choose an area from a mind map and formulate a SMART goal related to that area. Strategies and actions for achieving the goal are outlined, along with tips on overcoming obstacles.

The chapter also introduces the readiness to change graph, assessing the importance and confidence levels associated with making a change. The Eisenhower Matrix is introduced as a time management system, guiding readers on prioritising tasks and responsibilities.

Three Actions to Take:

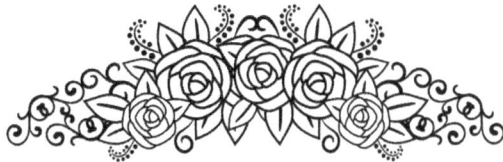

1. Draw your own mind map and write three SMART goals that are achievable in 3 months using the personal development coaching method.

2. Plot on the readiness to change graph where you currently are. Is there something you can do to increase your confidence or importance?

3. Use the time management Eisenhower Matrix to list your urgent and important actions to help you complete your goals.

Additional Information and Resources:

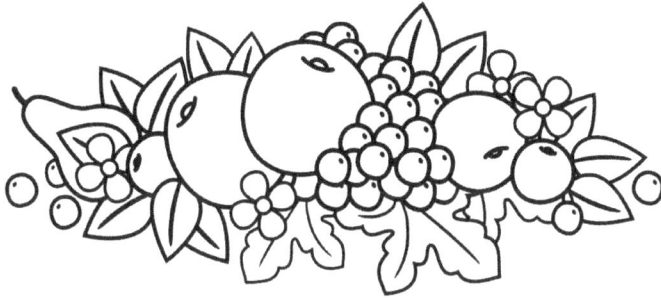

If you would like more information on any of this chapter, see the bonus offer 3 section for coaching resources towards the end of this book.

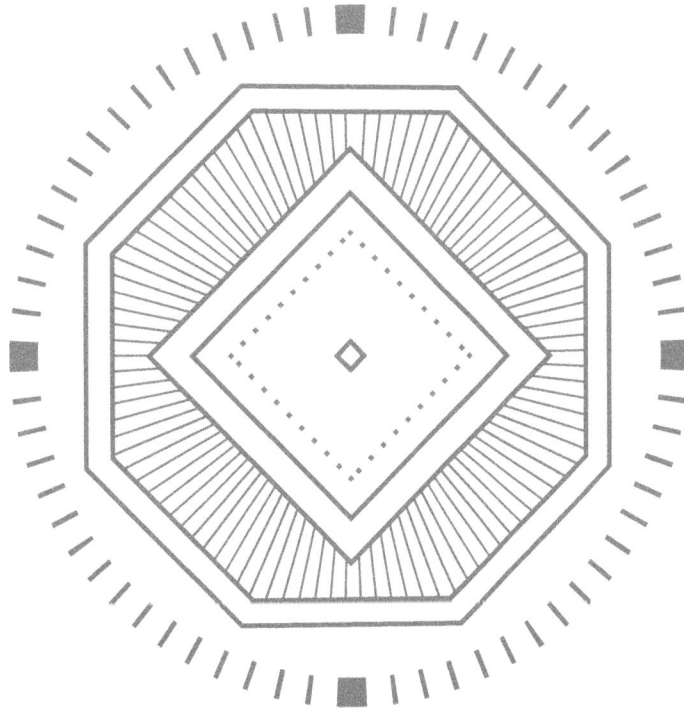

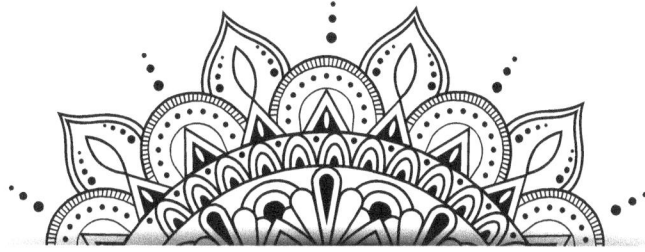

CHAPTER 6

Control Your Schemas

"One of my core beliefs is that belief itself is a choice that can be made of our own free will." (Steve Pavlina)

Do you ever find yourself engaging in repetitive patterns and questioning why, particularly when they appear to be self-defeating and dysfunctional?

It can be frustrating to say the least when we find ourselves in the same predicaments over and over. Schema therapy is about understanding early maladaptive schemas and modes and maladaptive coping styles which stem from early experiences and unmet core emotional needs.

The 18 early maladaptive schemas* represent recurring self-defeating core themes and patterns that persist across our lifetimes. Early schemas are linked to a child's fundamental emotional needs. When these needs go unfulfilled during childhood, schemas form, giving rise to unhealthy life patterns.

Schema therapy aims to assist individuals in fortifying their healthy adult mode, diminishing maladaptive coping modes, thereby reconnecting with their core needs and feelings. The therapy seeks to address and heal early maladaptive schemas, disrupting schema-driven life patterns and ultimately ensuring that individuals meet their core emotional needs in their daily lives. Schema therapy is a powerful tool to understand and change the deep-rooted beliefs and patterns that impact emotional wellbeing.

In this chapter, we will explore how you can start to recognise your schemas and express better ways to get your emotional needs met. It is not easy, but the benefits are worth it:

- Identify and challenge maladaptive beliefs and outdated patterns that may be hindering your mental wellness.
- Addressing and modifying any unproductive outdated schemas, you can change repetitive patterns and improve the chance of getting your core needs met.
- Insights into your thought patterns and behaviours, enhancing self-awareness.
- Taking control of your schemas empowering you to make meaningful changes in your life.
- Improved relationships as you gain a better understanding of your schemas, you can relate to others more effectively.

Research

Research shows that schemas developed in childhood can persist into adulthood and affect emotional well-being and life choices.

"Two roads diverged in a wood and I-I took the one less traveled by, and that has made all the difference." (Robert Frost)

Patterns that initially served as a functional means to fulfil our needs in early stages of life, may persist into adulthood. However, these patterns, initially a way to meet our emotional needs can become counterproductive in adulthood. In fact, they may hinder us from meeting our current emotional needs – such as difficulty trusting others, establishing healthy relationships, and feeling a sense of belonging.

Schema-focused therapy targets lifelong patterns by addressing negative cognitions deeply rooted in past experiences. This approach focusing on lifelong self-defeating patterns known as early maladaptive schemas.

What Constitutes an Early Maladaptive Schema?

Early maladaptive schemas are broad and pervasive themes or patterns about oneself and one's relationships, developed in childhood or adolescence, persisting, and reinforced throughout one's life and significantly dysfunctional according to Dr Jeffrey Young, who developed this model.

These schemas are highly stable and enduring, encompassing memories, bodily sensations, emotions, and cognitions. Once activated, they elicit intense emotions. For example, if someone has an early maladaptive schema related to **abandonment**, it includes memories of past abandonment, associated emotions like anxiety or depression, bodily sensations and thoughts anticipating people leaving them.

In essence, the early maladaptive schema represents the deepest level of cognition,

What Kinds of Early Childhood Experiences Contribute to the Development of Schemas?

This encompasses a child who faced unmet core needs, experiencing a deficiency in affection, empathy, or guidance. It may also pertain to a child who underwent trauma or victimisation by a dominating, abusive, or excessively critical parent or another person. Furthermore, a child who internalises parental voices, particularly those with punitive and condemning tones, can develop schemas. Alternatively, another circumstance arises when a child is exposed to an excess of positive influences, such as overprotection, overindulgence, or unrestricted freedom lacking appropriate boundaries.

Hence, early maladaptive schemas originate from experiences within our families or interactions with other children that caused harm. Whether it be abandonment, criticism, overprotection, emotional or physical abuse, exclusion, or deprivation, these experiences contribute to the development of schemas, becoming integral parts of our identity. Schemas essentially serve as valid reflections of early childhood encounters and act as **templates** for shaping and interpreting subsequent behaviours, thoughts, feelings, and relationships. Early maladaptive schemas encompass **ingrained** patterns of distorted **thinking**, disruptive **emotions,** and dysfunctional **behaviours**.

Indications that you may have an early maladaptive schema impacting your life include experiencing persistent challenges or feeling stuck in certain aspects you find difficult to change. Signs may manifest as feelings of inadequacy, loneliness, recurring depression, dependency on others, difficulties in selecting suitable partners, and being disconnected from your emotions. Chronic or lifelong presenting problems, such as eating disorders, substance abuse, recurrent depression and inflexible thinking and behavioural patterns, could also suggest

As they originate early in life, schemas become familiar and consequently, comfortable. To preserve the validity of our schemas, we may **distort** our perspective on life events. Schemas may remain inactive until triggered by situations pertinent to the specific schema. Schemas persist throughout one's life unless they are identified and modified, the first step is recognising them.

The 18 Early Maladaptive Schemas

Each of the 18 schemas signifies particular emotional needs that were insufficiently met in childhood or adolescence. (Young, 2007)

It may seem a little confusing if this is the first time you are hearing about schemas, but if you read or listen to the 18 listed below you may be able to identify some of your own schemas.

ABANDONMENT/INSTABILITY
The perceived lack of stability or dependability in those accessible for support and connection. This includes the belief that important individuals may be unable to consistently offer emotional support, connection, strength, or practical protection due to their emotional instability and unpredictability (e.g., displays of anger), unreliability, sporadic presence, imminent mortality, or the likelihood of abandoning the individual in favour of someone deemed better.

MISTRUST/ABUSE
The anticipation that others will cause harm, abuse, humiliate, deceive, lie, manipulate, or exploit. This typically entails the belief that the harm is deliberate or stems from unjustified and severe negligence. It may also involve the perception that one consistently ends up being treated unfairly compared to others or

EMOTIONAL DEPRIVATION

Anticipation that one's need for a standard level of emotional support will not be sufficiently fulfilled by others. The three primary forms of deprivation include:

Nurturance Deprivation: Lack of attention, affection, warmth, or companionship.
Empathy Deprivation: Absence of understanding, attentive listening, self-disclosure, or reciprocal sharing of feelings from others.
Protection Deprivation: Lack of strength, guidance, or direction from others.

DEFECTIVENESS/SHAME

The sense of being flawed, undesirable, unwanted, inferior, or invalid in significant aspects, or the belief that one would be unlovable if their true self were revealed to important individuals. This may encompass heightened sensitivity to criticism, rejection, and blame; self-consciousness; comparisons; and insecurity in the presence of others. It could also involve a feeling of shame regarding perceived flaws, which might be either private (such as selfishness, angry impulses, or unacceptable sexual desires) or public (for instance, an undesirable physical appearance or social awkwardness).

SOCIAL ISOLATION/ALIENATION

The sensation of being disconnected from the broader world, distinct from others, and/or not belonging to any group or community.

DEPENDENCE/INCOMPETENCE

The conviction that one lacks the capability to manage routine responsibilities competently without substantial assistance from others (e.g., self-care, problem-solving, exercising good judgment, undertaking new tasks, or making sound decisions). This often manifests as a sense of helplessness.

VULNERABILITY TO HARM OR ILLNESS

An intense apprehension that a sudden and disastrous event will occur imminently, and the belief that one cannot avert it. Concerns centre around one or more of the following:

Medical Catastrophes, such as heart attacks.
Emotional Catastrophes, like the fear of losing one's sanity.
External Catastrophes, for instance, concerns about elevators collapsing, falling victim to criminals, airplane crashes, or earthquakes.

ENMESHMENT/UNDEVELOPED SELF

Intense emotional engagement and proximity with one or more significant others (typically parents) to the detriment of complete individuation or typical social growth. This frequently entails the conviction that, without constant support from the other, at least one of the closely connected individuals cannot thrive or find happiness. It may also encompass sensations of feeling overwhelmed by or merged with others, or a lack of sufficient individual identity. Often, this experience is characterised by a sense of emptiness, confusion, a lack of direction, or, in extreme cases, questioning one's very existence.

FAILURE TO ACHIEVE

The certainty that one has experienced failure, is destined to fail, or is inherently inadequate compared to peers, particularly in realms of achievement such as academics, career, sports, etc. This frequently includes beliefs of being unintelligent, inept, untalented, ignorant, lower in status, or less successful than others.

ENTITLEMENT/GRANDIOSITY

The belief in one's superiority over others, entitlement to special rights and privileges, or exemption from the norms of reciprocity guiding typical social

pursue desires without consideration for realism, others' reasonable expectations, or the potential cost to others.

Alternatively, it may involve an exaggerated emphasis on superiority, such as striving to be among the most successful, famous, or wealthy, aimed at attaining power or control rather than seeking attention or approval. At times, it includes an excessive competitive attitude toward or domination of others, manifested through the imposition of power, enforcement of one's perspective, or control over others' behaviour without empathy or regard for their needs or feelings.

INSUFFICIENT SELF-CONTROL/SELF-DISCIPLINE

Widespread challenges or reluctance to employ adequate self-control and frustration tolerance in pursuit of personal goals, or to curb the excessive manifestation of emotions and impulses.

In its less severe manifestation, the individual exhibits an exaggerated focus on avoiding discomfort: steering clear of pain, conflict, confrontation, responsibility, or excessive effort – often to the detriment of personal fulfillment, commitment, or integrity.

SUBJUGATION

Excessive relinquishment of control to others due to a perceived sense of coercion, often driven by a desire to avoid anger, retaliation, or abandonment. The two primary forms of subjugation include:

Subjugation of Needs: Suppressing one's preferences, decisions, and desires.
Subjugation of Emotions: Suppressing the expression of emotions, particularly anger.

This typically involves the belief that one's own desires, opinions, and feelings

compliance, accompanied by heightened sensitivity to feeling trapped. This pattern often results in the accumulation of anger, leading to maladaptive symptoms such as passive-aggressive behaviour, uncontrolled temper outbursts, psychosomatic symptoms, withdrawal of affection, acting out, or substance abuse.

SELF-SACRIFICE

Excessive concentration on willingly fulfilling the needs of others in everyday situations, often at the cost of one's own satisfaction. The primary motivations include preventing others' distress, avoiding guilt associated with feeling selfish, or sustaining connections with individuals perceived as needy. This pattern frequently stems from a heightened sensitivity to others' pain and can occasionally result in the perception that one's own needs are inadequately addressed, leading to resentment towards those receiving care.

APPROVAL-SEEKING/RECOGNITION-SEEKING

An undue focus on seeking approval, recognition, or attention from others, or conforming to social norms, often at the cost of nurturing a secure and genuine sense of self. Esteem is predominantly reliant on others' reactions rather than one's own intrinsic tendencies.

This may involve an excessive emphasis on status, appearance, social acceptance, money, or achievement as avenues for gaining approval, admiration, or attention (not primarily for power or control). This pattern often leads to significant life decisions that are inauthentic or dissatisfying, as well as heightened sensitivity to rejection.

NEGATIVITY/PESSIMISM

A persistent and lifelong fixation on the negative facets of life, such as pain, death, loss, disappointment, betrayal, guilt, resentment, unsolved problems, and things that could go wrong. Simultaneously, there is a tendency to downplay or

This mindset often includes an overly heightened expectation, spanning various work, financial, or interpersonal scenarios, that things will eventually take a serious downturn or that positive elements in one's life will ultimately unravel. It typically entails an excessive fear of making mistakes that could lead to financial collapse, loss, humiliation, or being trapped in unfavourable situations.

Due to the exaggerated anticipation of negative outcomes, individuals with this mindset are frequently marked by chronic worry, vigilance, complaining, or indecision.

EMOTIONAL INHIBITION

Excessive restraint on impromptu action, emotion, or communication, typically aimed at sidestepping disapproval from others, feelings of shame, or the fear of losing control over one's impulses. The primary areas of inhibition encompass holding back anger and aggression; suppressing positive impulses, such as joy, affection, sexual excitement, or playfulness; encountering challenges in expressing vulnerability or freely communicating about one's feelings and needs; or placing an excessive emphasis on rationality while neglecting emotions.

UNRELENTING STANDARDS/HYPERCRITICALNESS

The inherent belief that one must continuously strive to meet exceedingly high internalised standards of behaviour and performance, usually to evade criticism. This often leads to feelings of pressure, difficulty in slowing down and a tendency towards hypercritical judgments of oneself and others. It is typically associated with significant impairment in experiencing pleasure, relaxation, maintaining good health, fostering self-esteem, achieving a sense of accomplishment, or forming satisfying relationships.

The unyielding standards commonly manifest as perfectionism, an excessive

the norm; establishment of rigid rules and 'shoulds' across various life domains, encompassing unrealistically high moral, ethical, cultural, or religious principles; or an obsession with time and efficiency, driven by the desire to accomplish more.

PUNITIVENESS
The belief that individuals ought to face severe punishment for their mistakes. This includes a disposition to exhibit anger, intolerance, a punitive attitude, and impatience toward those – oneself included – who fail to meet one's expectations or standards. Typically, it involves a challenge in forgiving mistakes, stemming from a hesitancy to consider extenuating circumstances, acknowledge human imperfection, or empathise with the feelings of oneself or others.

Schema Modes

Schema modes encompass the emotional states and **coping** responses that individuals undergo from moment to moment. Frequently, these modes are triggered by life situations to which we are particularly sensitive, referred to as our emotional buttons.

Many schema modes prompt us to overreact to situations or engage in behaviours that ultimately cause harm to ourselves. There are 10 identified schema modes, some are healthy, while others are maladaptive. They are grouped into four general categories:

- Child modes
- Maladaptive coping modes
- Maladaptive parent modes
- Healthy adult mode

CHILD MODES encompass experiencing, thinking, and behaving in a manner reminiscent of childhood.

Vulnerable child: experiences feelings of loneliness, isolation, sadness, misunderstanding, lack of support, inadequacy, deprivation, overwhelm, self-doubt, neediness, helplessness, hopelessness, fear, anxiety, worry, victimisation, worthlessness, lack of love, being unlovable, feeling lost, directionless, fragility, weakness, defeat, oppression, powerlessness, exclusion, being left out and pessimism.

Angry child: experiences intense anger, rage, fury, frustration, and impatience due to the unmet core emotional (or physical) needs of the vulnerable child.

Impulsive/undisciplined child: engages in selfish or uncontrolled actions based on non-core desires or impulses, struggling with the delay of short-term gratification. Often experiences intense anger, rage, fury, frustration, and impatience when these non-core desires or impulses cannot be fulfilled. May be perceived as spoilt.

Contented child: experiences feelings of being loved, content, connected, satisfied, fulfilled, protected, accepted, praised, worthwhile, nurtured, guided, understood, validated, self-confident, competent, appropriately autonomous, or self-reliant, safe, resilient, strong, in control, adaptable, included, optimistic and spontaneous.

MALADAPTIVE COPING MODES

Three broad coping styles that ultimately strengthen schemas by avoiding the experience of painful emotions linked to schema activation are:

- **Schema surrender** involves everything one does to perpetuate the schema

- **Schema avoidance** entails steering clear of situations triggering the schema or psychologically distancing oneself to avoid feeling the schema. An example is a person with a mistrust schema avoiding friendships due to the fear of being hurt or taken advantage of, reinforcing the belief when others sense the aloofness.
- **Schema overcompensation** involves excessively resisting the schema by doing the opposite of what it suggests. For instance, someone with a subjugation schema might rebel against those suppressing them. If overcompensation is too extreme, it can backfire and reinforce the schema.

As a result, we are left with one of the following:

Compliant surrenderer: behaves in a passive, subservient, submissive, approval-seeking, or self-deprecating manner in the presence of others due to a fear of conflict or rejection. Tolerates abuse and/or mistreatment, refrains from expressing healthy needs or desires to others, and engages in behaviour or selects people that directly perpetuates the self-defeating schema-driven pattern.

Detached protector: disconnects from needs and emotions, emotionally detaching from people and declining their assistance. Experiences withdrawal, spaciness, distraction, disconnection, depersonalisation, emptiness, or boredom. Engages in compulsive or excessive distracting, self-soothing, or self-stimulating activities. May adopt a cynical, aloof, or pessimistic stance to avoid investing in people or activities.

Over compensator: experiences and exhibits an excessively grandiose, aggressive, dominant, competitive, arrogant, haughty, condescending, devaluing, overcontrolled, controlling, rebellious, manipulative, exploitative, attention-seeking, or status-seeking demeanour. These feelings or behaviours initially develop as a means to

MALADAPTIVE PARENT MODES

Punitive parent: believes that oneself or others merit punishment or blame and frequently acts on these feelings by being accusatory, punitive, or abusive toward oneself (e.g., self-mutilation) or others. This mode pertains to the manner in which rules are enforced rather than the content of the rules themselves.

Demanding or critical parent: believes that the ideal way to be is to attain perfection or excel at a very high level, maintain order in everything, strive for high status, be humble, prioritise others' needs over one's own, or be efficient and avoid wasting time. Alternatively, the person may feel that it is incorrect to express feelings or act spontaneously. This mode is about the high standards and strict rules you have, not how you enforce them.

HEALTHY ADULT MODE

Healthy adult: nurtures, validates, and affirms the vulnerable child mode; establishes boundaries for the angry and impulsive child modes; encourages and supports the healthy child mode; counteracts and eventually supersedes the maladaptive coping modes; mitigates or moderates the maladaptive parent modes.

This mode also fulfills appropriate adult functions like working, parenting, assuming responsibility, and making commitments; engages in enjoyable adult activities; pursues intellectual, aesthetic, and cultural interests; maintains health; and participates in athletic activities.

Summary

Schema therapy delves into early maladaptive schemas, modes and maladaptive coping styles rooted in unmet core emotional needs from childhood. The 18 maladaptive schemas represent enduring self-defeating patterns.

Schema therapy aims to strengthen the healthy adult mode, diminish maladaptive coping, and address and heal early maladaptive schemas to disrupt harmful life patterns. Ultimately, the therapy helps individuals meet their core emotional needs and fosters emotional wellbeing.

Three Actions to Take:

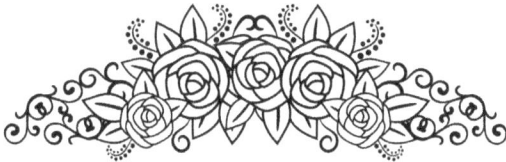

1. Identify any of the 18 maladaptive schemas you may have.

2. Start a schema journal (see next page) to help identify and analyse any patterns or schemas and their impact on your life. Use a non-judgemental curiosity to just notice any repeated themes that seem to be self-defeating.

3. Consider seeking professional guidance to assess and help shift any schemas toward the Healthy Adult mode.

Additional Information and Resources:

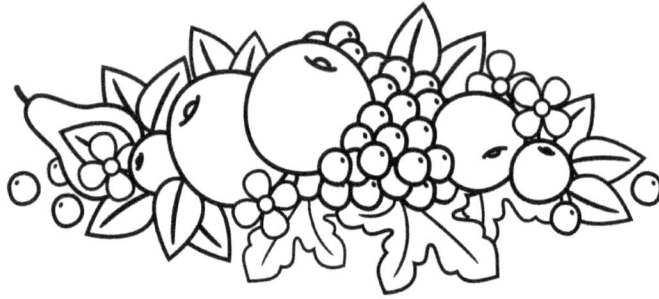

In the next chapter, we will delve deeper into the practical techniques and exercises that can help. If you find that your schemas significantly impact your daily life and wellbeing, consider consulting a qualified schema therapist for tailored support.

Schema Journal

The situation that impacted me ....

My feelings /emotions ....

My thoughts/reflections tied to emotions ....

My behaviour / actions ....

Which of the 18 early maladaptive schema patterns were triggered?........................

....

....

Which of the modes became active:

- o   Child (vulnerable/angry/impulsive) ....
- o   Parent (demanding / punitive) ....
- o   Coping (compliant surrender/ detached avoidant / over compensator)

Was my reaction excessive? ....

Were any of my cognitive distortions present (these were identified in Chapter 2)?
....

What would be a better balanced healthy adult response? ....

....

....

....

....

....

....

....

....

....

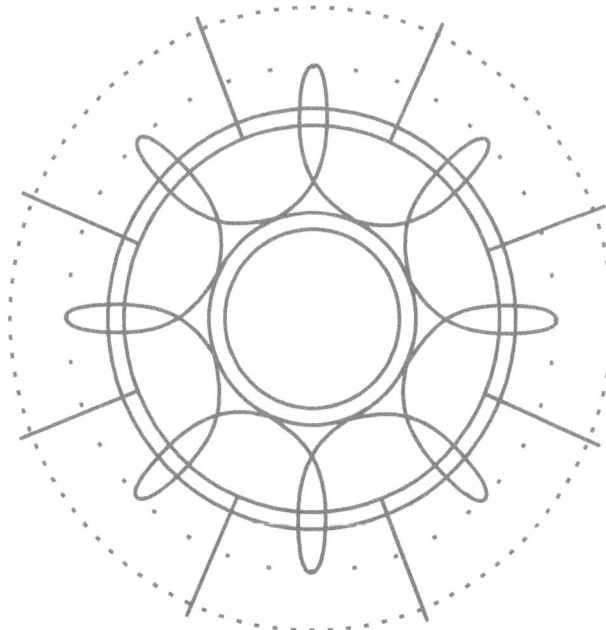

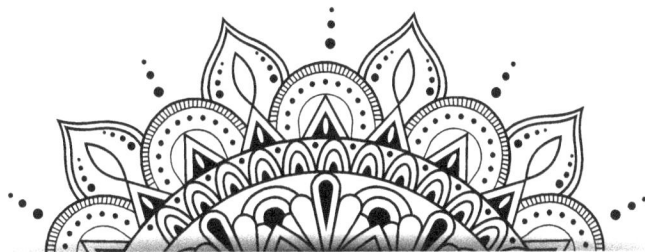

CHAPTER 7

Control Your Anxiety

"You don't have to control your thoughts. You just have to stop letting them control you." (Dan Millman)

Anxiety, with its persistent worry and overwhelming stress, can have a significant impact on your life. Due to anxiety being a response rooted in fear, fearing it and its symptoms can unfortunately intensify them. It becomes a self-fulfilling prophecy – you fear the anxious feelings and that fear triggers those same anxious feelings that you were trying to avoid in the first place.

However, the answer is not to avoid; instead, the answer is to acquire knowledge about your anxiety, treating it like a formidable opponent you aim to ally with. You see, anxiety is there to protect you and keep you safe from harm – sometimes it just does this too well and you miss out on exciting activities.

In this chapter, we will explore strategies to regain control over your anxiety by

- **Psychoeducation**: understanding the **physical** symptoms of anxiety can help you recognise and address them more effectively.
- **Fight or flight response:** exploring the fight-or-flight response with the guidance of experts like Dr Dan Siegel's hand model of the brain (2010), can help you understand and manage your anxiety better.
- **Breathing and progressive muscle relaxation (PMR)*:** learning breathing techniques and PMR can help you **regain control** over your **physiological** responses to anxiety.
- **Window of tolerance*:** learning about the window of tolerance can help you stay within your healthy range of **emotional arousal**.
- **Cognitive bias*:** identifying and addressing **cognitive biases** can improve your thought patterns and reduce anxiety. Similar to what we did in Chapter 2 improve your thinking.

Cognitive restructuring*: identifying and challenging negative thought patterns and beliefs. The goal is to replace irrational or harmful thoughts with more balanced and constructive ones. This technique aims to change dysfunctional cognitive habits, promoting healthier and more adaptive ways of thinking, which can, in turn, lead to changes in emotions and behaviours. It is commonly used to address anxiety.

Statistics

According to the World Health Organisation (WHO) last updated September 2023, Anxiety disorders are the world's most common mental disorders, over 300 million people are affected. Anxiety affects more woman than men. Anxiety symptoms frequently emerge in childhood or adolescence. There are highly effective treatments for anxiety disorders however only approximately 1 in 4

While occasional anxiety is a common experience, individuals grappling with anxiety disorders often endure heightened and excessive levels of fear and worry. These emotions are frequently accompanied by physical tension, as well as other behavioural and cognitive symptoms. Managing these intense feelings can be challenging, causing considerable distress, and persisting over an extended period if left untreated.

A Debilitating Illness

Anxiety disorders not only disrupt daily activities but also have the potential to negatively impact a person's family, social, academic and professional life.

Approximately 4% of the global population is currently estimated to be affected by an anxiety disorder. In 2019, a staggering 301 million individuals worldwide grappled with anxiety disorders, marking them as the most prevalent mental disorders by the World Health Organisation.

Despite the existence of highly effective treatments for anxiety disorders, a mere 27.6% of those in need receive any form of treatment, highlighting a significant treatment gap (World Health Organization, 2023). People may also experience more than one anxiety disorder at the same time. See the illustration of different types of anxieties that sit under the big umbrella term of anxiety.

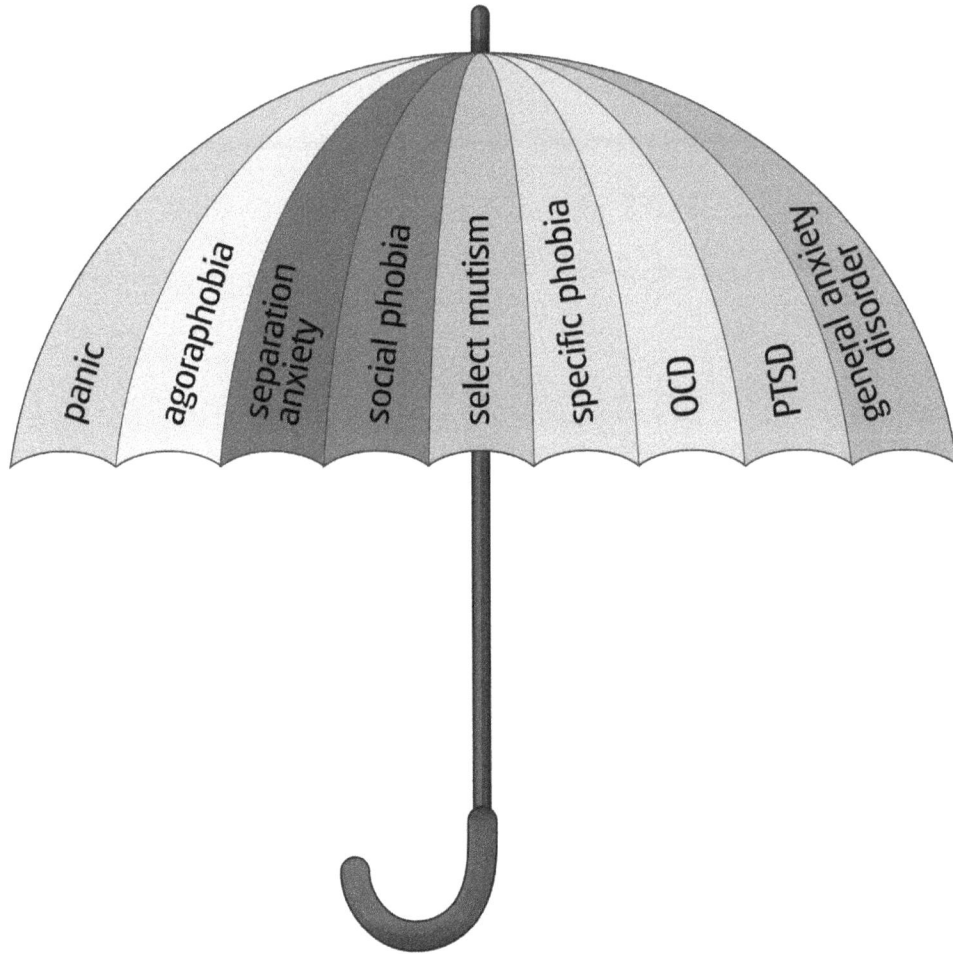

Different forms of anxiety that all sit under the big umbrella term of anxiety:

- **Generalised anxiety disorder (GAD):** persistent and excessive anxiety or worry about various life events and situations, often without a specific cause.
- **Panic disorder:** characterised by recurrent and unexpected panic attacks, which are sudden periods of intense fear or discomfort.
- **Agoraphobia:** an anxiety disorder involving a fear of situations or places where escape might be difficult or embarrassing, leading to avoidance of

- **Separation anxiety:** excessive fear or anxiety concerning separation from attachment figures, often experienced by children but can persist into adulthood.
- **Social phobia (Social Anxiety Disorder):** intense fear or anxiety related to social situations, leading to avoidance of social interactions.
- **Selective mutism:** consistent inability to speak in certain situations, such as social settings, despite speaking in other contexts.
- **Specific phobias:** intense and irrational fears of specific objects, situations, or activities, leading to avoidance and distress.
- **Obsessive-compulsive disorder (OCD):** characterised by intrusive thoughts (obsessions) and repetitive behaviours or mental acts (compulsions) performed to alleviate anxiety.
- **Post-traumatic stress disorder (PTSD):** occurs after exposure to a traumatic event and involves symptoms such as intrusive thoughts, nightmares, and avoidance behaviours. **Complex PTSD (C-PTSD):** a more severe and complex form of PTSD, often resulting from prolonged and repeated trauma, with additional symptoms such as difficulties in emotional regulation and interpersonal relationships.

According to the Australian Bureau of Statistics (2023), between 2020 and 2022, anxiety emerged as the prevalent category of mental disorders, affecting over 17.2 percent of Australians, which is more than one in six individuals.

The most prevalent comorbidity found among mental disorders was the coexistence of anxiety and affective disorders* – following closely was the association between anxiety disorders and substance abuse (Australian Bureau of Statistics, 2023).

The onset of anxiety disorders unfortunately, typically occurs early in life. This is why it is important to provide early intervention. I typically work with young

If you suspect Post-Traumatic Stress Disorder (PTSD)*, it is recommended to seek professional advice from your GP and allied health professional. PTSD is a mental health condition that can develop in individuals who have experienced or witnessed a traumatic event. Symptoms may include flashbacks, nightmares, severe anxiety, and uncontrollable thoughts about the event, persisting beyond the initial trauma.

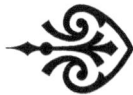

Safety Warning: If you have concerns for your safety or someone else's it is crucial to seek professional advice with a GP or closest Emergency Department.

Complex PTSD* (C-PTSD) is a psychological condition stemming from prolonged exposure to severe and repeated trauma, involving difficulties in emotional regulation, interpersonal relationships, and self-perception. While I have effectively treated these disorders, it would be naive of me to believe that a journal book could provide significant assistance without the backing of a medical and allied health team.

Effective treatments exist to help support you manage this condition. Several organisations offer targeted support, First Responders Support Hub, Open Arms Veterans and Families and Reach-out Australia. (*Please see the Help Organisations section at the end of this book for more information*).

Common concerns and protests to learning to control anxiety, usually stem from the comfort of avoiding whatever is feared or causing the anxiety.

"Anxiety is just a part of who I am; there's no way to control it."

My response: While anxiety may be a part of your life, you can learn strategies

"I've tried to control my anxiety before, but nothing works."

My response: What works for one person may not work for another. This chapter explores multiple techniques, giving you the opportunity to discover what helps you personally.

"I'm afraid that trying to control my anxiety will make it worse."

My response: The right strategies can help you manage your anxiety without making it worse. This chapter aims to provide you with a toolkit to control your anxiety more effectively.

"If you know the enemy and know yourself, you need not fear the result of a hundred battles." (Sun Tzu, The Art of War)

Psychoeducation to Tame the Beast

Other words commonly used to describe anxiety are worry, nervousness, tension, apprehension, uneasiness, fear, dread, restlessness, jitters, concern, shyness, and stress.

These feelings are all connected to anticipating something negative. Anxiety exists to ensure your survival, keeping you safe from harm and enhancing your performance, it is referred to as the fight or flight response.

Anxiety primarily triggers this fight or flight response to either confront the perceived threat (fight) or escape from it (flight), and animals share this instinct. So, you can see anxiety isn't all negative; it can keep you safe and even be beneficial

Anxiety can be used to motivate you by creating a sense of urgency or concern, prompting individuals to take action or make changes to address the source of their anxiety.

For example, studying for an upcoming test, or maintaining a healthy lifestyle after having a health scare. This motivation can lead to problem-solving and proactive behaviours aimed at reducing stress and achieving goals.

Mr Potato Head

Anyone who has been in to see me about anxiety usually gets Mr Potato Head drawn for them – see illustration. I use this simplified picture to show the physiological reactions to anxiety. Understanding what your body is doing and why can help you feel like you are back in control.

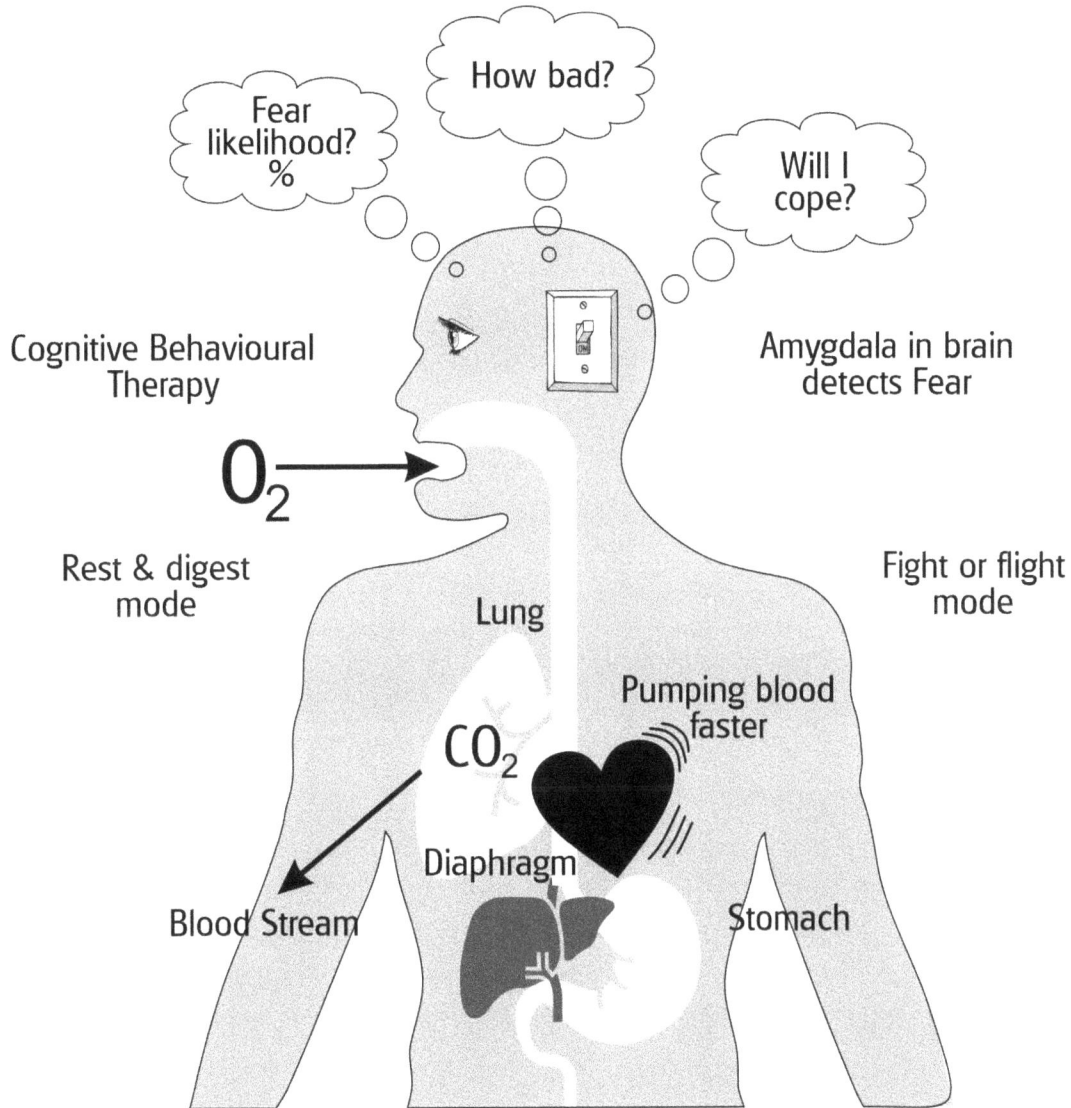

Our brain perceives a threatening situation and, in an instant a cognitive appraisal is performed, and the amygdala turns on, (just like a binary light switch). Our body begins the fight or flight response, priming our bodies ready to either attack the perceived threat or get away from it. Most people remember how anxiety feels because it is quite intense, the heart starts beating fast to pump blood to muscles around the body in order to deal with the threat. Our breathing can become rapid and shallow (called hyperventilation) which causes oxygen and carbon dioxide levels to become unbalanced, effecting our blood pH. Your body knows what to do to regulate and restore the blood pH, however you will most likely experience more physical symptoms like dizziness, tingling and light headiness.

Psych tip: I find slow deep diaphragm belly breathing is so underrated! Practicing this technique can help you prevent hyperventilation from occurring or at least minimise the effects. There are instructions for this later in the chapter, including an audio.

Pupils dilate so you may experience changes to your vision, muscles tense ready for fight or flight and can sometimes shake and tremble. The bronchioles in our lungs open up, our liver releases glucose and our digestion slows which can cause a dry mouth, nausea, or butterflies in our tummy. We now have a heightened alertness to assess the situation. These physiological changes prepare the body for a rapid and efficient response to a perceived threat in order to keep us alive.

While this response is crucial for survival in acute situations, sometimes the anxiety is caused by a feared situation that you cannot fight or flee from, for example an embarrassing situation, public speaking, or fear of failure. The fight and flight response typically doesn't assist in these situations. It's crucial to comprehend the cognitive assessments made by our brain so that we can modify our thinking in these contexts. Furthermore, chronic activation due to ongoing stressors can have negative effects

The Challenge Journal ✳ Katrina Langhorn

There are three parts to anxiety: your **thoughts**, your **body,** and your **actions**.

Sometimes the first we are aware of is the physical symptoms we **feel** in our body.

Thoughts (Cognitive)	Body (Physical)	Actions (behavioural)
Anticipating a negative outcome and overlooking alternative possibilities can trigger anxiety, starting as an insistent worrisome thought. These include unrealistic thoughts, beliefs, and expectations.	Your heart rate rises, muscles tense, and breathing quickens, boosting mental alertness – these changes ready your body for action.	Feeling a desire to escape or react strongly, you might avoid anxiety-inducing situations, preventing yourself from engaging in enjoyable activities.

The goal is to reduce anxiety to a manageable level, enabling the positive effects like increased energy and motivation for significant tasks – while minimising drawbacks such as missed opportunities, difficulties in making friends, or challenges in school or work.

The goal is not to completely eradicate all anxiety because it is there as a survival instinct, the goal is to reduce anxiety, so it is more in your control, rather than it controlling you. Some of the ways we can manage anxiety are:

Thoughts (Cognitive)	Body (Physical)	Actions (behavioural)
• Cognitive restructuring • Realistic thinking • Detective thinking	• Deep belly diaphragmatic breathing • Progressive muscle relaxation (PMR)	• Worry scale or subjective units of distress (SUDS) • Exposure not avoidance • Hierarchy ladders

The stress response can be reduced by consciously breathing using the diaphragm. Abdominal breathing helps to control the nervous system and encourages the body to relax, bringing about a range of health benefits (referred to as rest and digest).

Deep Belly (Diaphragmatic) Breathing

- Find a comfortable spot to sit or lie down.
- Ease your shoulders down away from your ears.
- Place one hand on your stomach and the other on your chest.
- Inhale through your nose gently,
- Taking in air until you can't anymore.
- Observe the air entering your abdomen, expanding your stomach to push out and make your belly extend,
- Try to keep your chest steady as you only want the air to pass down your chest but not be stored there because you want it lower into your diaphragm.
- Then purse your lips, as if sipping through a straw. Exhale slowly through your lips until you have exhausted all of your breath, feeling your stomach

- Repeat these steps several times for the best results. You may feel lightheaded this is normal, do not worry- just try to relax until you are ready to stand up.

Psych tip: *I practice my deep breathing often throughout the day even when I don't need it, this way when I do need it, I have enough muscle memory that my parasympathetic nervous system knows what I am doing and cooperates.*

Access to this recording:
https://www.atfullpotential.com.au/the-challenge-journal

Progressive Muscle Relaxation

To engage in progressive muscle relaxation, allocate approximately 15 minutes for this calming exercise.

- Choose a tranquil setting where interruptions are unlikely.
- Sit comfortably with a straight back and your feet flat on the floor.
- Close your eyes or lower your gaze, practicing breathing for five minutes from the above deep belly breathing instructions.
- Then sequentially tense specific muscle groups for ten seconds, then release and completely relax them for ten seconds.
- Be attentive to the distinct opposite sensations of tension and relaxation.

Psych tip: *Do NOT hold your breath; we are briefly holding the tension in our muscles but not holding our breathing – breath normally during step 1-6.*

- Start by tightening your biceps and curl both fists, as if lifting weights. Hold muscles tense for ten seconds, then release and relax for 10 seconds.
- Wrinkle your forehead and facial muscles, purse your lips, press your tongue against the roof of your mouth, and hunch your shoulders. Hold for 10 seconds, then relax for 10 seconds.
- Arch your back while taking a deep breath into your chest. Hold tension (not breath) for 10 seconds, then release and relax for another 10 seconds.
- Inhale deeply and gently push out your stomach. Hold for 10 seconds, (not breath) then relax for 10 seconds.
- Point your feet and toes downward, tightening your shins. Hold for 10 seconds, then release and relax for 10 seconds.
- Simultaneously pull your toes backwards and tighten your calves, thighs, and buttocks. Hold for 10 seconds, then relax for 10 seconds.
- Conclude by closing your eyes and practicing deep belly breathing like above for another five minutes. Afterward, resume your normal activities with a calm and relaxed manner.

The Worry Scale or Subjective Units of Distress (SUDS)

Having a common method to gauge your anxiety levels and effectively communicate them to others can be advantageous for everyone's comprehension. It also proves valuable for monitoring progress and improvement. It is simply a scale between 0 and 10; 0 being relaxed and 10 being extremely anxious.

Connecting Thoughts with Emotions

Anxiety arises from our thoughts, and to address these anxious thoughts, it is

instances of anxiety by noting the situation, our thoughts, emotions, and actions. Utilising a worry scale can also help express the level of anxiety experienced in each situation.

Situation:

What happened?.........................*e.g., I have a speech tomorrow*
What did I think?........................e.g., *I will mess it up*
How did I feel?...........................e.g., *nervous*

What is my worry (SUD) level?   0   1   2   3   4   5   **6**   7   8   9   10

What was my behaviour/action? ....*e.g., stay awake thinking about it for hours*

Expressing these thoughts in writing can be beneficial because our thoughts are often fast and automatic, making them easy to overlook. It is easy to fall into the trap of associating a situation with negative feelings, leading to the belief that avoidance is a solution. However, this avoidance strategy is not effective in the long run. While it may temporarily reduce anxiety, it doesn't address the underlying issue.

Simply avoiding situations doesn't contribute to genuine learning or coping. Unfortunately, anxiety tends to **generalise**, meaning avoidance can expand from specific places to a broader range of environments. For example, avoiding a large shopping centre may become avoiding all types of shops including petrol stations.

Slowing down this process and identifying the thoughts that are associated with a situation and the feeling requires **practice**. Journaling can assist this process.

Cognitive Restructuring – Realistic Thinking

Unrealistic thinking perpetuates anxiety, marked by an exaggerated belief in the likelihood and consequences of negative events, along with accepting unrealistic automatic thoughts without scrutiny or challenging them. So anxious thoughts, beliefs and expectations need to be **identified**, then they can be **challenged** with evidence so a more **realistic** thought can develop.

Two cognitive distortions that we tend to over evaluate:

The outcome probability bias* refers to an individual's inclination to overestimate the chances of an anticipated negative result. Overestimating, the likelihood of unpleasant events – inflating the probability of a negative outcome (expressed as a percentage %). This is the first thought bubble depicted In the illustration of Mr Potato head.

In my experience, many people tend to make this 100 %, as if the negative event has already taken place! Whilst we are such smart cognitive creatures this is where we may be too smart for our own good. We can imagine all sorts of awful events that are painful like embarrassing (messing up during public speaking), or rejection (going for a promotion and not being successful). It is better to gather evidence and put a more realistic % on the likelihood of the feared event occurring. For example, fearing your plane will crash.

Reality: the likelihood of airplane crashing is extremely low. Well below 1 in a million. Commercial airplanes undergo rigorous testing, maintenance, and safety regulations to ensure the structural integrity of the aircraft. Catastrophic failures of this nature are exceedingly rare and are designed to be prevented through stringent engineering standards and continuous monitoring. Air travel remains one of the safest modes of transportation globally.

Another cognitive distortion that we tend to over evaluate is overestimating the severity of the consequences if the event does occur, leading to catastrophic thinking. Whilst embarrassment is not a preferable outcome you don't die from it. The fight and flight response is designed to protect your safety and your life. This is the second thought bubble depicted in the illustration of Mr Potato Head.

For more realistic thinking about the severity of messing up during public speaking, what is the worst that can happen? You mess up, you forget your lines? Will people laugh? Probably, is it the end of the world? NO, it will be okay. Will you cope? Of course you will. Has it happened to other people before? You betcha!

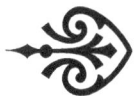

Safety Warning: When anxiety is due to a **real actual threat** it is important to keep you safe so don't try to use cognitive restructuring for those cases.

Realistic thinking is kind of like being a **detective** and looking for **clues** to change the worried thoughts, beliefs, and expectations. Like before where we identified the situation, and what you thought, how you felt and rated on the worry SUDS scale, now we add gathering your **evidence**.

Has it happened before? How many times? What is the best that could happen? Are you jumping to conclusions – what is the actual probability in %? What else could happen? What happens to other people in this situation? What skills do you have to cope with this situation? What would you think if it happened to someone else? How will this look in two weeks, two months, two years' time? How will you cope if it does happen?

Situation:

What happened?..

What did I think?..

How did I feel?...

What is my SUD level   0   1   2   3   4   5   6   7   8   9   10

What is the **evidence**?...

....

What is a **calmer realistic thought** instead? ....

What is my SUD level now?   0   1   2   3   4   5   6   7   8   9   10

Upon uncovering realistic thoughts, it is essential to actively incorporate them. This involves consciously **choosing** to think realistic thoughts during challenging situations, which can be difficult and requires **practice** (there is more space to journal at the end of this chapter).

Initially, realistic thoughts may feel unfamiliar, while anxious thoughts may seem quicker, more intense, and automatic. However, through practice and experience, you will come to realise that the realistic thoughts are **more accurate** and beneficial.

With consistent practice, realistic thinking gradually becomes automatic, gradually replacing the old anxious thoughts. In these instances, **thought cue cards*** can be beneficial, offering alternative, more constructive thoughts and questions derived from your journal entries for common anxiety-inducing situations, at least until your realistic thinking replaces anxious thoughts.

"I must not fear. Fear is the mind-killer. Fear is the little-death that brings total obliteration. I will face my fear. I will permit it to pass over me and through me. And when it has gone past I will turn the inner eye to see its path. Where the fear has gone there will be nothing. Only I will remain." (Frank Herbert, Dune)

Fight Fear by Facing Fear

Exposure is the opposite of avoidance and avoidance in the long run does not help. Fight fear by facing your fears!

Graded exposure* is a therapeutic technique that involves gradual and systematic exposure to anxiety-inducing stimuli or situations. It is used to help individuals overcome fears and anxiety by incrementally facing and **adapting** to the feared stimuli in a **controlled manner**. We do this by using an agreed hierarchy ladder system with SUDS rating to help achieve goals (using rewards for motivation if necessary).

Exposure and Response prevention* means staying in the situation long enough and often enough for the anxiety to subside and for you to realise that nothing bad will happen, or if it does, you find that you will cope.

Exposure and Response prevention is a therapeutic strategy used in behaviour therapy – particularly in the treatment of anxiety disorders and compulsive behaviours. It involves deliberately interrupting the typical behavioural response that reinforces or maintains an undesired behaviour. This approach aims to break the association between the triggering stimulus and the response, ultimately reducing or eliminating the problematic behaviour.

Hierarchy ladder*

Set a practical fear goal e.g., *to attend a big popular festival like the Easter show or comic com or a music concert.*

What is the worried thought? e.g., *I will get lost, I might vomit on a ride*

List other situations that provoke similar fear *e.g., going to large shopping centres, attend small school fete, going on small rides with friends, going on long bus/car/train rides.*

Now, rate each on the SUDS scale and place the number on the ladder:

The ladder may look like this:

	10	To attend a festival like Easter show
High harder steps	8	Go to large shopping centres
Medium steps	6	
		Go on small rides with friends
	4	
Low easier steps	2	Attend small school fete
	0	Go on long bus/car/train rides

These steps can be completed multiple times in multiple different places, with multiple different people e.g., parents, friends. Each step is a reward (even if that reward is praising yourself for being brave). Utilise the detective thinking during each exposure so you can gather firsthand evidence – either the bad fear doesn't happen or if it does that you can cope! It is time to progress up the ladder to the next steps once exposure has occurred enough times, and where SUDS are re-rated around a Level 2 or reduced by 50%.

Summary

Symptoms commonly initiate in childhood or adolescence and persist into adulthood. There is a higher likelihood for girls and women to encounter anxiety disorders compared to boys and men.

There are different types of anxiety disorders that all sit under the umbrella term of Anxiety.

The distinction lies in whether you are dominated by your anxiety or have control over it, for example, being *controlled by* your anxiety or being *in control of it*.

You have the power to manage and control your anxiety rather than letting it define your life. The transformation lies in being under the influence of your anxiety versus having the ability to manage and control it.

Three Actions to Take:

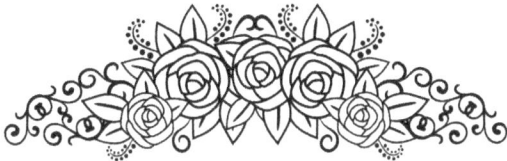

1. Practice deep breathing exercises and progressive muscle relaxation to manage your physiological responses to anxiety.

2. Connect thoughts with feelings:

Situation:

What happened? ....
What did I think?..
How did I feel?..
What is my SUD level?   0   1   2   3   4   5   6   7   8   9   10
What was my action? ....

3. Identify and challenge cognitive biases and irrational thoughts that contribute to your anxiety:

Situation:

What happened? ....
What did I think?...
How did I feel?...
What is my SUD level?   0   1   2   3   4   5   6   7   8   9   10
What is the **evidence**? ....
....
What is a calmer realistic thought instead? ....
What is my SUD level now?   0   1   2   3   4   5   6   7   8   9   10

....
....
....
....
....
....
....

Additional Information and Resources:

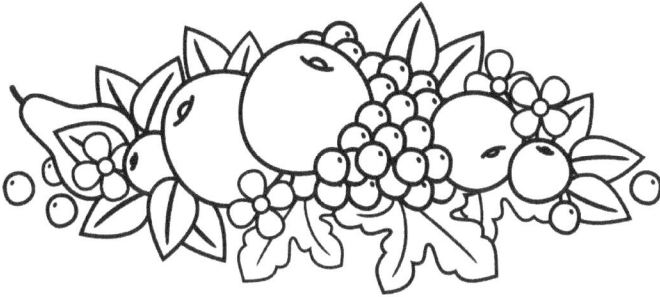

In the next chapter, we will delve into practical exercises and techniques to further help you control your anxiety. If your anxiety significantly impacts your daily life, consider seeking guidance from a qualified therapist or counsellor who specialises in anxiety management.

Another option is to undertake online cognitive behavioural therapy e-CBT. This can be done over the internet in your own time and comfort. See the bonus offer 3 section and Help organisations towards the end of this book.

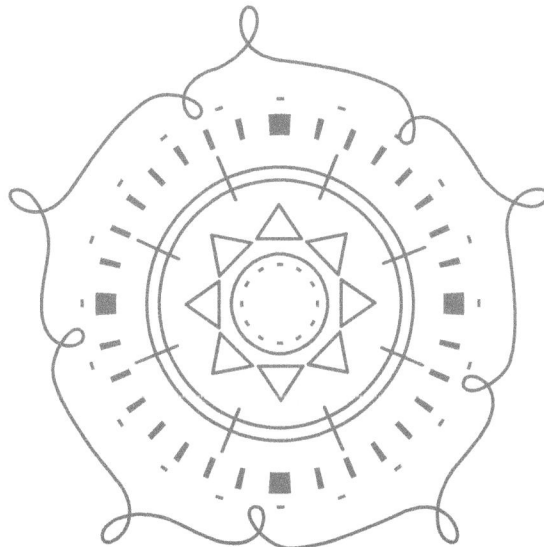

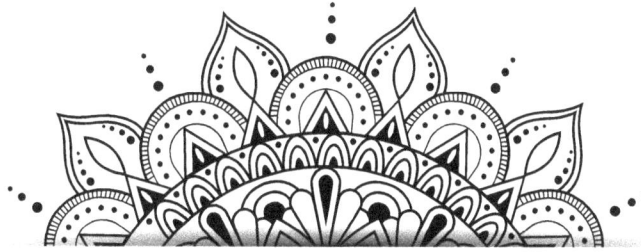

CHAPTER 8

Relax Your Mind

"Mindfulness is a form of mental activity that trains the mind to become aware of awareness itself and to pay attention to one's own intention."
(Dr Daniel Siegel)

In a fast-paced world filled with constant distractions and demands, the practice of mindfulness offers a path to inner peace, presence, and self-awareness. This chapter delves into the profound realm of mindfulness and its transformative power in:

- **Reducing stress:** mindfulness helps in managing stress, promoting relaxation, and enhancing overall wellbeing.
- **Improving focus:** it sharpens your concentration, making you more efficient in your tasks.
- **Enhancing emotional regulation:** mindfulness equips you to handle emotions with grace and resilience.
- **Enhancing self-awareness:** it deepens your understanding of yourself,

- **Better relationships:** mindfulness fosters better communication and empathy, enriching your interactions with others.

A book called *Stolen Focus, Why You Can't Pay Attention* (2022), explores a broad spectrum of factors contributing to a singular issue: the diminishing ability to focus. In Hari's book it categorises the myriad of reasons behind our attention deficits into two primary groups: excess and deficiency (or too much and too little). These include an overflow of information, stress, heightened surveillance and manipulation and the prevalence of ADHD diagnoses.

Our ability to pay attention is collapsing. The decline in our attention span is evident. In this book, Hari suggests the reasons behind this phenomenon and recommends ways to reclaim our focus. He describes 12 factors that have been substantiated to diminish individuals' attention spans and notably, many of these factors have seen an upsurge over the past few decades, at times significantly.

Having conversations with numerous teenagers, including my own two, has led me to an ongoing disagreement: they believe they can engage in multiple forms of media simultaneously – even while studying! Neuroscientists delved into this and observed that when people think they are multitasking, they are essentially juggling tasks.

The constant switching between activities incurs a cost, known as the switch-cost effect*, resulting in a decline in performance. Research revealed that those who received text messages and stopped to read them performed, on average, 20% worse (Hari, 2022).

Once a week, I would enter a correctional facility, leaving my smartphone, watch and laptop behind. Engaging in singular tasks without interruptions, I operated noticeable improvement in my attention span while it was not having to constantly switch between juggling tasks.

The Alternative

Have you ever observed that during routine tasks like vacuuming, folding laundry, or driving (when you know the way because you drive it often), your mind tends to wander off?

You get engrossed in thoughts about various matters such as daydreaming about a vacation, fretting over an upcoming event, or pondering numerous trivial things like how pandas get so fat eating only bamboo?

In such instances, your focus is not on the present experience, and you feel somewhat disconnected from the current moment. This state of operating is commonly known as **automatic** pilot mode. Mindfulness, on the other hand, stands in contrast to automatic pilot mode. It involves fully immersing oneself in the present moment, also known as the **being** mode. This approach provides a means to break free from automatic and unproductive thought patterns, allowing one to be genuinely present rather than dwelling on the past or worrying about the future.

The distinction lies between living on autopilot, constantly swept up in thoughts of the past and future or being fully present in the here and now, with all your senses engaged. It is mindful – not mind full!

"The present moment is the only moment available to us, and it is the door to all moments." (Thich Nhat Hanh)

By cultivating a more frequent state of mindfulness, one can establish a new habit that effectively undermines old, unconstructive, and automatic thought patterns. For individuals grappling with emotional challenges, these entrenched habits may revolve around excessive fixation on the future, dwelling on the past, or engaging in negative self-reflection.

In such cases, the objective of mindfulness training is not control, elimination, or resolution of these distressing experiences. Instead, it strives to hone a skill that positions individuals better to resist or disengage from these unproductive habits that contribute to distress and hinder positive action.

The primary aspect of mindfulness entails witnessing your experiences through a more sensory perception mode – rather than engaging in analytical thinking mode. The innate inclination of the mind is to analyse rather than fully experience something directly. Mindfulness seeks to redirect one's attention from the realm of thoughts to the act of simply observing thoughts, emotions, and bodily sensations – such as with the five far senses of touch, sight, sound, smell, and taste – with a gentle and inquisitive curiosity.

This can be done by a simple grounding activity: just become aware of what you are touching e.g., bottom on seat, feet on floor, what you can see around you, what sounds can you hear, what smells are around you and what can you taste? e.g., toothpaste? coffee?

A mentor suggested that I try to have a mindful coffee each morning, smelling the brew, listening to the espresso machine, looking lovingly at my coffee mug with uplifting phrases, sipping, and savouring the taste… Luckily, while feeling the coffee in my mouth, I discovered a crunchy, abnormal texture – had it of been a day on autopilot I probably would have just drunk the coffee none the wiser –

Exploring this facet of mindfulness involves paying attention to the intricate particulars of your observations. Similar to the coffee example above, what if you were to observe an object like a strawberry?

Think of the mindful exploration to articulate its visual aspects – its appearance, shape, colour, and texture. You may employ descriptive terms such as red, bumpy, or small.

This same approach is applicable to emotions, where descriptors like burdensome, tedious, or stressed can be used to characterise and understand the nuances of the emotional experience, expanding your emotional repertoire and suspending judgement.

Embracing an accepting attitude toward your experiences is crucial.

Prolonged emotional distress often arises from efforts to evade or manipulate these experiences. In mindfulness, there is no endeavour to pass judgment on experiences as good or bad, right, or wrong. The approach does not involve an immediate need to control or avoid experiences; instead, acknowledging all aspects of one's experience proves to be one of the most demanding aspects of mindfulness.

Developing this nonjudgemental perspective requires time and consistent practice. Approaching one's experiences with a kind and gentle curiosity is a means of fostering a nonjudgemental practice.

A key objective of mindfulness is to engage wholeheartedly to enable yourself to encompass the entirety of your experience without overlooking any elements. Strive to observe all facets of the task or activity at hand, engaging in it with complete care and undivided attention. This appears to be increasingly challenging for us due to the world of multitasking, mobile phones ringing and dinging, the

When attentively observing your own experiences, a degree of effort is necessary to concentrate on one thing at a time, continuously, from moment to moment.

Distractions and wandering thoughts naturally arise during observation, tempting one to pursue them with further contemplation. The essence of being present lies in cultivating the ability to recognise when you have transitioned from observation and sensing mode to thinking mode. When this shift occurs, it's okay – just simply acknowledge it and guide yourself back to focusing on one single task.

When I practice yoga, I try to stay focused on the poses e.g., sun salutation or warrior, as well as my breathing. However, often my mind wanders... *Have I remembered all the sequence? Am I doing downward-facing dog pose correctly? Are others looking at me in amusement?* Then I remember just to be present and breathe while holding the position.

Mindfulness encompasses a range of techniques, including meditation as well as other practices:

- **Meditation:** traditional mindfulness meditation involves focusing attention on the breath, a mantra, or an aspect of the present moment. This practice helps cultivate awareness and a sense of calm.
- **Mindful Breathing:** similar to meditation but focuses solely on your breath. During a formal dedicated session which pays attention to each inhalation and exhalation, bringing your awareness to the sensations of breathing. During yoga practice, for example when focus is placed on the breathing.
- **Body Scan:** progressively focus on different parts of your body, paying attention to sensations, tension, or relaxation. This helps increase awareness of physical sensations.

- **Mindful Walking:** take a slow, deliberate walk, paying attention to each step, the sensation of movement and the environment around you. It's a way to bring mindfulness into daily activities.
- **Mindful Eating:** eat slowly and savour each bite. Pay attention to the taste, texture, and sensation of the food. This practice encourages a deeper connection with your eating experience. This is what I was doing with the strawberry and the coffee-swimming cockroach!
- **Mindful Listening:** fully engage in the act of listening without formulating responses in your mind. Be present with the sounds around you, whether it is nature, music, or people talking.
- **Gratitude Practice:** focus on aspects of your life that you are grateful for. Regularly acknowledging and appreciating positive aspects can foster a more positive outlook.
- **Mindful Journaling:** write down your thoughts and feelings without judgment in this journal. This practice helps in self-reflection and gaining insight into your experiences.
- **Visualisation:** imagine a peaceful scene or engage in guided imagery to promote relaxation and focus. Visualisation can help reduce stress and anxiety.
- **Mindful Activities:** engage in routine activities with full attention, such as washing dishes, gardening, or cleaning. Approach these tasks as opportunities for mindfulness.
- **Loving-Kindness Meditation:** directing positive and compassionate thoughts toward yourself and others. This practice aims to cultivate feelings of love and kindness.
- **Breath Awareness in Daily Life:** bring awareness to your breath in various situations throughout the day, not just during formal meditation sessions. This can be particularly helpful during moments of stress.

Remember, mindfulness is about being present and fully engaged in the current moment, and these are just a few examples of the various ways to incorporate this practice into your daily life.

Window of Tolerance

A concept in psychology that refers to an optimal range of arousal or activation levels within which an individual can effectively process information and respond to stressors. When a person is within their window of tolerance, they can manage challenges and emotions in a balanced manner. However, if arousal levels become too high (hyperarousal) or too low (hypoarousal), individuals may experience difficulties in coping with stress and regulating their emotions.

This concept is often applied in the context of trauma and stress-related disorders to understand and support emotional regulation.

Imagine a child who has had a challenging morning; they had a fight on the bus to school and had also forgotten to bring their lunch. By the afternoon lesson on wind powered experimental vehicles, they were unable to concentrate and follow the instructions to complete the task successfully. Then, they become uncharacteristically frustrated with the rest of the class that seemed to enjoy the lesson.

This is a scenario where the child might be outside their window of tolerance. The accumulated stressors from the day have pushed them beyond their optimal range of emotional arousal, unable to take in new learning and resulting in a reaction that is more intense and less regulated than what might be typical for them. Sometimes it just takes time to reset, something to eat and a good night's sleep for example.

Practicing mindfulness can also help **expand** our window of tolerance by promoting awareness of emotions in the present moment. This heightened awareness enables us to adeptly navigate challenging emotions and enhances our ability to withstand life's difficulties. Consistent mindfulness practice contributes to improved emotion regulation, making it easier to manage and respond effectively to various emotional experiences.

Some common complaints I often hear in response to mindful exercises:

"I don't have time for mindfulness."

My response: Mindfulness does not demand hours of your day. Even dedicating a few minutes to mindful practices can create a positive impact on your well-being. I often suggest when you are time poor to just start off utilising the time when we are waiting for something, time not used for anything else. For example, breath awareness in the supermarket waiting in line or even during an advert on the television.

"Mindfulness seems too spiritual or 'way out there' for me."

My response: mindfulness is a practical and evidence-based approach, rooted in psychology. It is about focusing your attention on the present moment, making it accessible to everyone, regardless of their spiritual beliefs.

"I've tried mindfulness before, but it didn't work for me."

My response: mindfulness is a skill that requires practice and patience. Like any skill, it improves with time and commitment. Keep trying and you will likely experience its benefits.

*"Do not dwell in the past, do not dream of the future,
concentrate the mind on the present moment."* (Buddha)

Visualisation or Guided Imagery

Visualisation* and guided imagery* are terms that are often used interchangeably, and their distinctions can be subtle. However, some nuances exist in their usage:

- Visualisation can be a self-directed process where individuals create mental images independently. It may not necessarily involve external guidance or structured scripts.
- Guided imagery unlike visualisation, involves external guidance. This can come in the form of a live instructor, therapist, or a recorded audio script. The purpose is to lead the individual through a specific experience or scenario.

A fundamental approach to utilising imagery for relaxation involves closing your eyes and envisioning yourself in a serene and soothing place. This place could be a real location from your past experiences, or a fictional setting crafted in your mind. It might be a serene beach, a cosy fireplace, a shaded spot in the woods, or any other peaceful environment that brings you comfort. Engage all your senses in your imaginative journey – see the waves gently caressing the shore, the dappled light through the leaves, hear the birdsong, or the leaves rustling. Inhale the fragrance of flowers, grass, or the salty sea air and sense the sun's warmth or the gentle breeze on your skin. Allow yourself to truly feel present in that moment. A natural smile can accompany a relaxed body as you enjoy this mental escape for a few minutes.

Example of Guided Imagery & recording:

This guided relaxation exercise involves closing your eyes, taking slow, deep breaths, and imagining a tranquil garden. Picture yourself strolling along a serene path, entering a peaceful sanctuary filled with your favourite elements. Engage your senses in exploring textures, sounds, and fragrances, fostering deep relaxation. When ready, return to the present with a sense of contentment, knowing you can revisit this peaceful sanctuary whenever needed. Open your eyes, stretch, and resume your day with a refreshed and alert state of being.

✸ **Access to this recording:**
https://www.atfullpotential.com.au/the-challenge-journal

Here is a step-by-step guide on cultivating mindfulness and incorporating it into your daily life:

Recognising Automatic Pilot Mode:
- Acknowledge instances where your mind tends to wander during routine or boring tasks that don't require much of your attention. An example of operating on autopilot is apparent when comparing the focused attention required during initial driving lessons to the ease and familiarity of driving after three decades of experience.
- Identify moments of daydreaming, future worries, or past pondering that disconnect you from the present. Sometimes this can occur when our head hits the pillow, and you want to sleep but your brain decides to dissect all the interactions of your day.

Understanding Mindfulness:
- Differentiate between automatic pilot mode and mindfulness.
- Embrace mindfulness as the practice of immersing yourself fully in the present moment, in the NOW.

Breaking Unproductive Thought Patterns:
- Cultivate a frequent state of mindfulness to establish a new, constructive habit. This will help break some of the old more unhelpful thinking habits.
- Recognise and undermine old, automatic thought patterns that contribute to emotional distress. Replacing the old habits with the new helpful habits.

Mindfulness for Emotional Challenges:
- Manage emotional challenges by taking a moment to delay the urge for immediate control or elimination.
- Develop skills to resist unproductive habits and promote positive actions.

Sensory Perception in Mindfulness:
- Focus on sensory perception rather than analytical thinking.
- Redirect attention from thoughts to the observation of thoughts, emotions, and bodily sensations.
- Engage the five senses (touch, sight, sound, smell, and taste) with gentle curiosity.

Practical Mindfulness Exercise:
- Conduct a quick sensory activity: recognise what you are touching, seeing, hearing, smelling, and tasting.
- Apply this awareness to immerse yourself in the present moment.

Detailed Observation:
- Pay attention to intricate details when observing objects or emotions.
- Articulate visual aspects and employ descriptive terms to understand and characterise experiences.

Embracing Wholehearted Engagement:
- Enable yourself to encompass the entirety of your experience.
- Observe all facets of tasks with complete care and undivided attention.

Coping with Distractions:
- Acknowledge the challenge of multitasking in a digital world.
- Consider limiting external interruptions to enhance focus and participation.

Acceptance and Nonjudgmental Perspective:
- Embrace an accepting attitude toward experiences without passing immediate judgments.
- Understand that prolonged distress may arise from attempts to manipulate or evade experiences.

Transition between Observation and Thinking Mode:
- Acknowledge the shift from observation to thinking mode without judgment.
- Gently guide yourself back to focusing on one task at a time when distractions occur.

Exploring Mindfulness Techniques:
Explore various mindfulness techniques beyond meditation, refer back to this list of 12 techniques and use what resonates with you.

Remember:
- Mindfulness is about being fully present and engaged in the current moment. I suggest regularly engaging in the simple five senses approach.
- Choose techniques that resonate with you and incorporate them into your daily life gradually, like mindful coffee in the morning – minus the cockroach, of course!
- By following these steps and incorporating mindfulness techniques, you can cultivate a more mindful and present way of living in the NOW.

Summary

Mindfulness is the practice of paying deliberate and non-judgmental attention to the present moment. It involves observing your thoughts, feelings, and bodily sensations without trying to change or fix them.

Observing everyday tasks reveals a common tendency for the mind to wander, preoccupied with thoughts unrelated to the present moment. This automatic pilot mode, prevalent in our multitasking digital age, disconnects us from the current experience.

Mindfulness, in contrast, encourages immersion in the present, termed the being mode. Developing this practice involves accepting experiences without judgment, acknowledging distractions, and returning focus. Mindfulness techniques extend beyond meditation and include mindful breathing, body scans, mindful walking, and mindful eating.

Embracing gratitude, journaling, visualisation, and loving-kindness meditation are

each moment, fostering a nonjudgmental perspective and a skilful focus on one task at a time.

> *"Mindfulness isn't difficult; we just need to remember to do it."*
> (Sharon Salzberg)

Three Actions to Take:

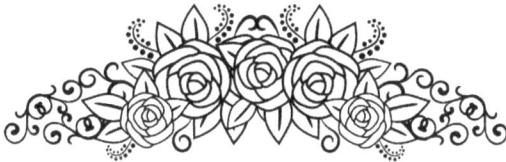

1. Set aside a few minutes each day to practice mindfulness, starting with simple techniques like breath awareness, or mindful walking even if it is just from parking your car and walking into work/school/shop or your mailbox or even just from the bedroom to the kitchen. Practice a quick sensory activity: recognise and name what you are touching, seeing, hearing, smelling, and tasting. Apply this awareness to immerse yourself in the present moment in the right NOW.

2. Use the guided imagery audio, use often to help relax your mind.

3. Understand that mindfulness is a skill that develops with consistency and patience, and its benefits become more evident over time. An easy way to start the practice is to write a gratitude journal. Use the space provided to start you off.

Additional Information and Resources:

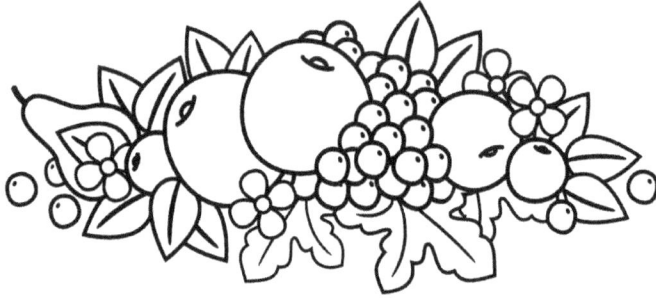

Explore further resources and techniques to deepen your mindfulness practice, such as meditation apps, books, or classes.

In the next chapter, we will delve into practical exercises and tips for incorporating mindfulness into your daily life to help with stress. If you have specific questions or concerns about practicing mindfulness, consider seeking guidance from a mindfulness instructor, yoga teacher or therapist who can provide tailored support.

Gratitude Journal

What are you doing right now? ....
....
....

Name what you are touching, seeing, hearing, smelling, and tasting.............................
....
....
....

What are you most grateful for today? ....

....
....
....

What are other things that you are grateful for? ....
....
....
....
....
....
....
....
....
....
....

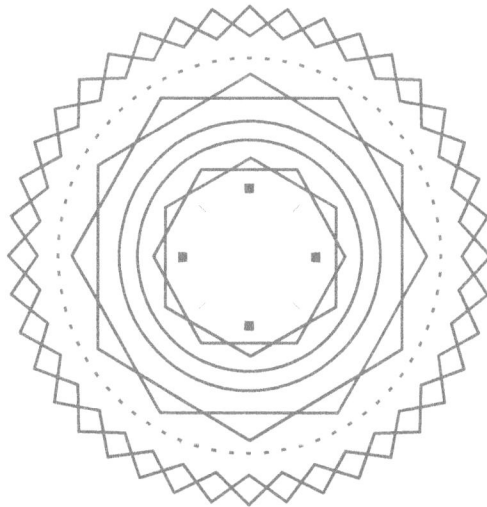

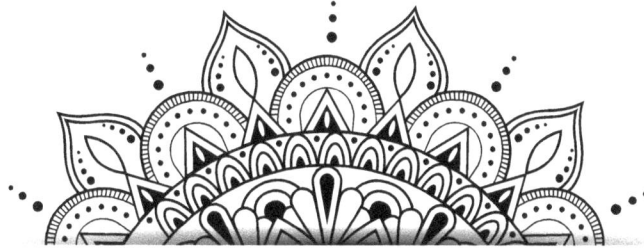

CHAPTER 9

Manage Your Stress

"Everything can be taken from a man but one thing: the last of the human freedoms-to choose one's attitude in any given set of circumstances, to choose one's own way." (Viktor E Frankl)

Stress management is an essential skill for navigating the challenges of modern life. In this chapter, we will explore effective strategies to help you manage stress and regain control over your well-being. Stress management is a critical skill in today's fast-paced world, and this is your guide to understanding and effectively managing the stress that life throws your way.

Benefits:

- **Improved physical health:** effective stress management can reduce the risk of stress-related health problems, such as heart disease and high

- **Enhanced emotional wellbeing:** stress management techniques can help reduce anxiety and depression, promoting emotional resilience.
- **Better relationships:** managing your stress can lead to improved communication and healthier relationships with others.
- **Increased productivity:** reducing stress can boost your focus and productivity.
- **Enhanced quality of life:** overall, stress management can lead to a higher quality of life, with more joy and fulfillment.

The Shocking Truth:

Chronic stress can lead to various health issues, including a weakened immune system, making you more susceptible to illnesses.

The prevalence of morbidity and mortality resulting from stress-related illnesses is concerning. Emotional stress significantly contributes to the top six causes of death in the USA, including cancer, heart disease, accidental injuries, respiratory disorders, cirrhosis of the liver, and suicide. According to data from the U.K approximately 180,000 individuals succumb to various forms of stress-related illnesses annually states Salleh. (2008)

The difference is in how you react to stress. You can either let it overwhelm you, leading to negative health consequences, or you can master it through effective management.

Stress management is the process of employing various techniques and strategies to cope with, reduce, or eliminate stressors in your life. It involves recognising your stressors, developing effective coping mechanisms, and taking steps to minimise stress's impact on your physical and mental health.

Inadequately managed stress, particularly when it becomes overwhelming, can result in fatigue, psychological disorders such as depression, anxiety, and insomnia, as well as various health issues like a compromised immune system.

The prevalence of stress is alarming. The *Australian Psychological Society* found as many as 35% of Australians acknowledging significant stress. (Australian Psychological Society, 2015)

75% of adults in America were found to be experiencing moderate to high levels of stress scholars Anderson et al., found in 2015.

A similar survey a year earlier found stress is also a significant concern for teenagers, and if left unaddressed, it may lead to serious long-term health consequences. (Breckler & Ballard, 2014).

Selye (1974) defined stress as the body's nonspecific response to any demand placed on it. Stressors, the stimuli triggering stress responses, can be external (e.g., major life changes, unpredictable events, social demands) or internal (e.g., personal fears, uncertainty, perfectionistic expectations).

Acute stress arises from recent or anticipated stressors, while chronic stress results from prolonged exposure to unrelenting demands. Different individuals respond to stressors based on their type, nature, and subjective interpretation. Various stress models, one of which is the General Adaptation Syndrome* (GAS), helps to better comprehend the nature of the stress response.

In the General Adaptation Syndrome (GAS) model, Selye (1974) proposed that different stressors trigger a common physiological response. The model has three phases: alarm, resistance, and exhaustion.

- During the alarm phase, the body reacts to a stressor with increased energy (the fight or flight response).
- The resistance phase involves the body staying alert, releasing cortisol to handle the stressor until it's resolved, or the body can't resist anymore.
- In the exhaustion phase, prolonged or intense stress depletes energy reserves, potentially leaving the body vulnerable to illness. The GAS model explains how the body responds to stressors.

Encountering stress and acute stress is inevitable as we navigate life's demands. (MacDonald, 2003)

It is important to note that not all stress is necessarily negative. Eustress*, a term introduced by Selye and later defined by Lazarus (1966), refers to positive stress when a stressor is viewed as a challenge. The Yerkes-Dodson curve suggests that moderate stress can enhance performance until an optimal level is reached. At this point, stressors are seen as manageable challenges.

However, some situations lead to negative stress responses or distress, where stressors are perceived as threats. According to the Yerkes-Dodson curve, performance may decline when stress levels surpass the optimal point. Beyond this, stressors can be overwhelming, causing individuals to question their ability to cope.

Optimal
Peak

BUFFERS
1. SLEEP
2. NUTRITION
3. EXERCISE

STRONG

Productivity / Performance

Increasing
Alertness

Increasing
Anxiety

EUSTRESS
Motivational good
stress

Calm

Distress

WEAK

Bored

Burnout

LOW   Level of Stress / Arousal   HIGH

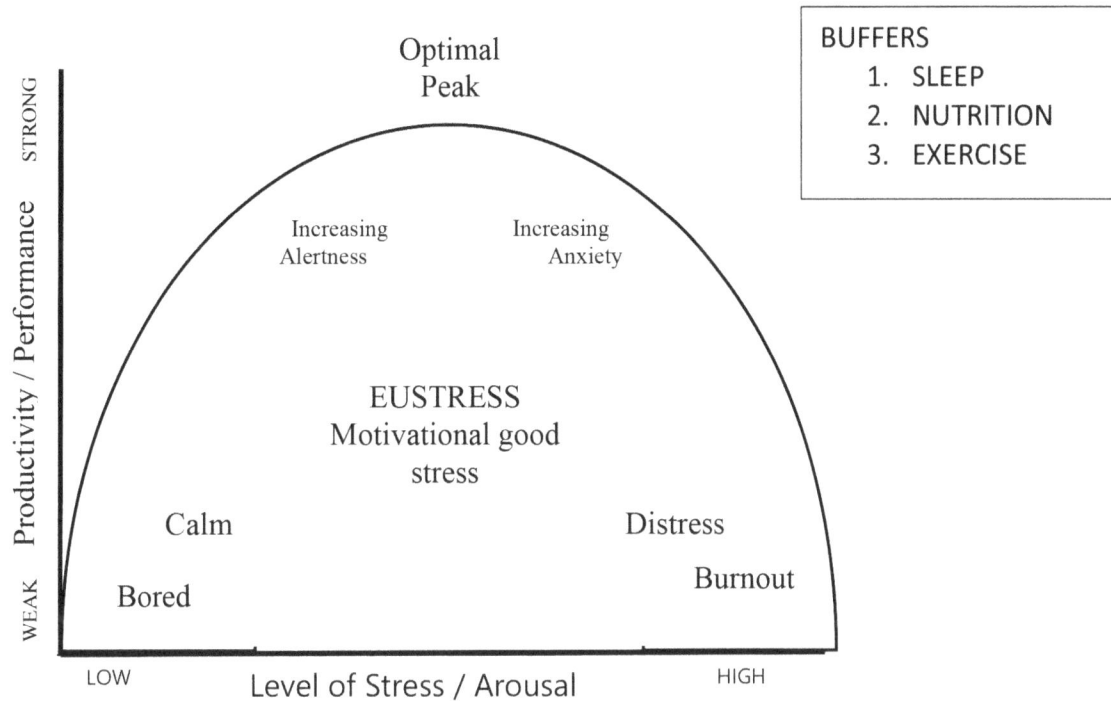

The Yerkes-Dodson Stress Curve illustrates the relationship between your stress and your performance. It shows that there is an optimal level of stress that enhances your performance and too much or too little stress can have detrimental effects. This curve is an oldie but a goodie, possibly more relevant today than it was in 1908 when it was first described by Yerkes and Dodson. The graph illustrates the interaction of stress on performance.

When stress is low (on the left of horizontal x axis) the productivity is also low (sub-level) to the persons potential, motivation is not high, and procrastination can occur, the persons arousal is underwhelmed. Alternatively, on the right of the horizontal x axis when stress is high the productivity has already peaked and is declining, this is when a person is in distress and is overwhelmed.

The Yerkes-Dodson Law is a psychological principle that describes the relationship between arousal (or stress) and performance. The law suggests that there is an optimal level of stress for peak performance, and both low and high levels of stress can result in decreased performance.

Here is an explanation of the Yerkes-Dodson graph:

Curve:
- This graph is typically represented as an inverted U-shaped curve.
- The X-axis represents the level of arousal or stress (ranging from low to high).
- The Y-axis represents performance.

Low Arousal/Stress:
- On the left side of the curve (low stress), performance is relatively low.
- When individuals are not aroused enough, they might lack the motivation or alertness needed to reach their optimal performance.

Optimal Arousal/Stress:
- As stress increases towards the middle of the curve, performance improves.
- There is an optimal level of stress where individuals are sufficiently motivated and alert, leading to their peak performance.

High Arousal/Stress:
- However, as arousal continues to increase beyond the optimal point, performance starts to decline.
- Too much stress or arousal can lead to anxiety, distraction, or impaired decision-making, negatively affecting performance.

In summary, the Yerkes-Dodson Law suggests that there is an optimal level of stress for peak performance. Too little or too much stress can result in suboptimal performance. The ideal level of arousal may vary for different tasks and individuals.

This concept has been widely applied in fields such as sports psychology, education, and work performance to understand and optimise performance under different levels of stress.

The goal is to stay balanced around the middle in optimal performance with just enough stress to be motivated but not too stressed that you are overwhelmed, the Goldilocks Principle.

There are three protective buffers that can help the individual be resilient against the detrimental stress responses and remain at their individualistic full potential. These healthy helpful protective buffers are sleep/rest/relaxation, nutrients, and water (I also include a digital diet for my clients) and exercise/activity.

The Yerkes-Dodson Law, along with the influence of protective factors like **sleep**, **nutrition,** and **exercise**, on wellbeing and performance, finds support in a substantial body of research spanning various fields. Here are some key studies and findings related to each aspect:

Protective Buffer of Sleep:

- **Cognitive Performance:** Sleep has a profound impact on cognitive performance. Research published in the journal, *Sleep*, highlighted the importance of sleep for memory consolidation and cognitive functions, emphasising the role of both quantity and quality of sleep. (Watson et

- **Arousal and Emotional Regulation:** Sleep is also crucial for emotional regulation. Studies have shown that sleep deprivation can lead to heightened emotional reactivity and decreased ability to regulate emotions.

Protective Buffer of Nutrition:

- **Brain Function:** Nutrition plays a vital role in brain function. For instance, omega-3 fatty acids found in fish have been associated with cognitive performance, and a balanced diet that includes a variety of nutrients supports overall brain health.
- **Mood and Mental Health:** Research in the field of nutritional psychiatry suggests that diet can influence mood and mental health. For example, a study published in 2017 found an association between a healthy diet and a reduced risk of depressive symptoms by Marx, Moseley, Berk and Jacka. (2017)

In the journal *Nutrients* (Du et al., 2021) results suggest a connection between inferior dietary habits and increased perceived stress, diminished sleep quality, and reduced resilience.

Protective Buffer of Exercise:

- **Cognitive Benefits:** Numerous studies have demonstrated the cognitive benefits of exercise. For example, a review published in the British Journal of Sports Medicine in 2018 found that aerobic exercise has positive effects on cognitive function, including attention, memory, and processing speed.

- **Mood Regulation:** Exercise has been shown to have mood-regulating effects. The release of endorphins during physical activity can contribute to improved mood and reduced stress levels.

It is widely acknowledged that engaging in physical exercise is among the most effective methods for coping with stress. According to the Stress in America survey, 43% of adults highlighted exercise as their chosen stress management strategy. Many individuals reported experiencing positive outcomes such as improved mood, a more positive self-concept, and reduced stress levels through regular exercise. (Breckler & Ballard, 2014)

Many studies show the positive effect that exercise has on stress reduction, one study in *Health Psychology* in 1992 examined the hypothesis that a single session of aerobic exercise can act as a protective factor against psychosocial stress responses in women.

The findings demonstrated that exercise mitigates bio measured reactivity to psychosocial stress. Moreover, compared to the attention placebo control, exercise reduced the occurrence and intensity of anxiety-related thoughts associated with anticipating interpersonal threats and challenges. (Rejeski et al., 1992)

I have also noticed that over the last two decades, when someone's stress is affected by time constraints, there is a perilous mistake of stealing time from one of the three protective factors.

For example, if you have a deadline, you may skip the gym or yoga class, you may drink more caffeine and have sugary snacks, which can also affect your sleep. It then becomes a much quicker slippery slope away from your optimal performance and plummets into crash and burn. Try not to steal from those three protective

lifestyle. Another way is to use a time management system, so you do not get crushed under stressful time constraints.

Eisenhower Matrix, you may recall we used this in *Chapter 5*'s Goal Setting, and it can be useful here to help manage stress.

> *"The key is not to prioritize what's on your schedule,*
> *but to schedule your priorities."*
> (Stephen Covey)

Some common difficulties I hear from people during discussions on managing stress:

"I don't have time to manage my stress."

My response: Stress management doesn't require extensive time commitment. In fact, it can improve your efficiency and overall quality of life.

"I've tried stress management methods before, but they didn't work."

My response: different stress management techniques work for different people. We'll explore a variety of approaches to help you find what suits you best.

Using Techniques from Previous Chapters to Manage Stress:

Mindfulness and meditation practices serve as tools to anchor you in the present, diminishing the influence of future anxieties and past remorse. Engaging in these

wellness. Regular mindfulness sessions contribute to maintaining tranquillity amidst stress, fostering an overall sense of wellbeing.

Progressive Muscle Relaxation (PMR) is commonly employed as a complementary approach in stress management, anxiety reduction and the enhancement of overall wellbeing. In addition to the previous PMR script there is also an alternate script and audio in *Chapter 10*.

Use Eustress from the Yerkes-Dodson Stress Curve as motivation and direct your energy. Positive Eustress evokes excitement and enhances performance because it is perceived as manageable within your coping capabilities.

How Harnessing Eustress Helped my Journey

Between completing my psychology honours degree and embarking on my teaching master's program, I enrolled in a TAFE course focused on teaching adult learners. I thoroughly enjoyed the course and held great admiration for my instructor, who exemplified the virtues of an excellent teacher for adult learners. As the semester approached its end, I planned an overseas trip to Europe and Türkiye.

In a rush to complete my last assignment and hand it in before the trip, it was unexpectedly rejected. I was instructed to resubmit because it was below par.

"Well, I never!" as my nanna would say.

Although I outwardly felt upset and indignant, these emotions were merely masking the disappointment I harboured within myself. Determined to prove the rejection wrong, I channelled all my eustress, along with a hint of anger into my

aimed to achieve – to bring out the effort she knew I could produce. She was pure brilliance, and I will never forget that lesson.

Harness eustress to reach your full potential.

Use the protective buffers of **sleep** (rest/relaxation/meditation), **nutrition** (hydration) and **exercise** to buffer against the onslaught of stress and keep you at your optimal performance.

Sleep hygiene* refers to a set of practices and habits that are conducive to getting good quality sleep on a regular basis. These practices aim to promote a healthy sleep pattern and improve overall sleep quality. Sleep hygiene encompasses various lifestyle and environmental factors that can affect sleep, and adopting good sleep hygiene can help individuals establish a consistent and restful sleep routine. Some common elements of sleep hygiene include:

Consistent sleep schedule: going to bed and waking up at the same time every day, even on weekends, helps regulate the body's internal clock. My son adopted this early in life and I have seen no one ace this any better than he has.

- **Comfortable sleep environment:** creating a comfortable and conducive sleep environment involves having a comfortable mattress and pillows, controlling room temperature, and minimising noise and light.
- **Limiting stimulants:** avoiding stimulants like caffeine and nicotine close to bedtime can help improve sleep quality.
- **Establishing a bedtime routine:** engaging in relaxing activities before bedtime, such as reading or taking a warm bath, can signal to the body that it's time to wind down.
- **Limiting screen time:** exposure to the blue light emitted by electronic

of the sleep hormone melatonin. It's recommended to limit screen time before bedtime.

- **Regular exercise:** engaging in regular physical activity can promote better sleep, but intense exercise close to bedtime should be avoided.
- **Managing stress:** developing effective stress management techniques, such as mindfulness or meditation, can help reduce anxiety and promote relaxation before bedtime.
- **Watch diet before bed:** avoiding heavy meals close to bedtime and opting for a light snack if hungry can be beneficial. Also, staying hydrated is important, but excessive fluids before bedtime may lead to disruptions to the bathroom.
- **Limiting naps:** while short naps can be refreshing, long or irregular napping during the day may interfere with night-time sleep.

By incorporating these practices into one's daily routine, individuals can optimise their sleep hygiene and enhance the likelihood of experiencing restful and rejuvenating sleep.

Summary

The Yerkes-Dodson Law is typically represented as an inverted U-shaped curve. It describes the relationship between stress and performance. According to this law, performance increases with arousal or stress up to a certain point, after which it starts to decline. It illustrates the idea that there is an optimal level of arousal for peak performance, and deviations from this optimal point can lead to suboptimal outcomes.

The Eisenhower Matrix is a time management tool that categorises tasks into

and stress reduction. Mindfulness and meditation practices help individuals stay present, minimising the impact of future concerns and past regrets, leading to stress management and improved mental well-being.

PMR is a relaxation technique involving systematic muscle tension and relaxation, guided to reduce physical tension, enhance relaxation, and promote overall wellbeing, often utilised in stress and anxiety management.

Three Actions to Take:

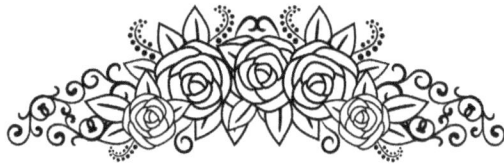

1. Assess your current stress levels and identify specific stressors in your life. Place yourself on the Yerkes Dodson curve:

    - Are you at your optimum level?
    - Can you harness eustress to help motivate you?
    - Are you stealing from the three protective factors?

    If sleep is affected, try the sleep hygiene to see if that can assist you.

2. Use progressive muscle relaxation, when we are stressed, we don't always recognise that we are tensing our muscles. In the next chapter there is an audio available.

3. Revisit *Chapter 5* for Eisenhower Matrix and *Chapter 8* for mindfulness

Additional Information and Resources:

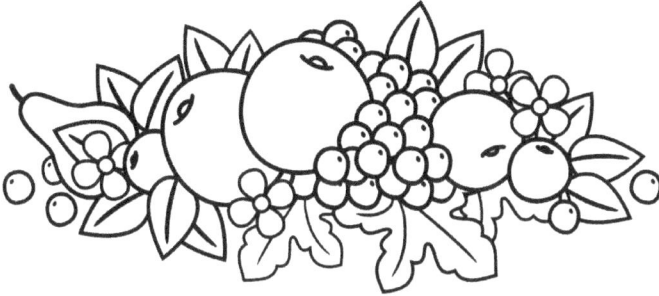

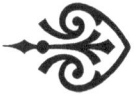

Safety Warning: *PTSD is a condition that requires health professionals, this chapter on managing stress, may be helpful but it is not enough to treat PTSD. PTSD is an anxiety disorder, not just a reaction to normal everyday stress.*

If you are struggling with severe stress or anxiety, consider seeking professional guidance from a therapist or counsellor to assist your specific needs.

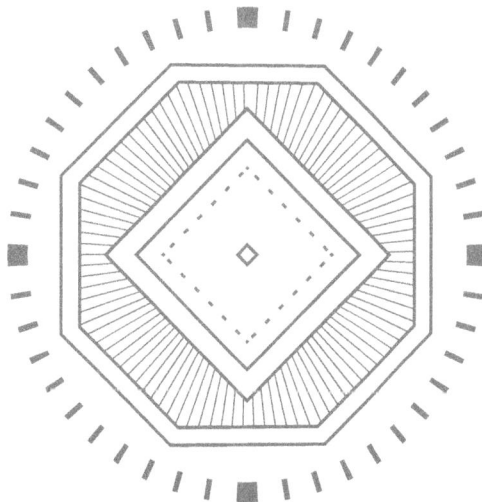

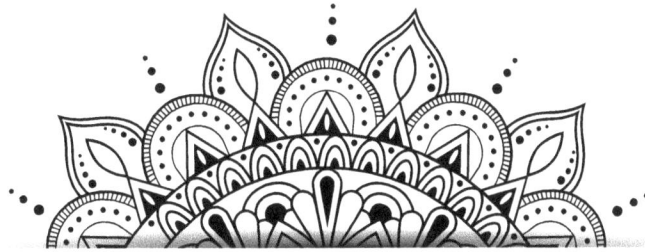

CHAPTER 10

Manage Your Anger

"Anybody can become angry - that is easy, but to be angry with the right person and to the right degree and at the right time and for the right purpose, and in the right way - that is not within everybody's power and is not easy." (Aristotle)

Anger is a universal emotion, neither 'right' nor 'wrong.' However, it is our **response** to anger that can make a significant difference in our lives and the lives of others.

Experiencing anger can be challenging, yet it is a common and natural emotion that everyone encounters. Anger is often considered a secondary emotion, serving as a protective mechanism or a cover-up to mask other more vulnerable feelings. This tendency arises because anger is socially acceptable and easier to express. However, emotions lying beneath anger may be intricate and less straightforward to recognise, acknowledge, or talk about.

While we may believe we are simply angry, there is often a complex blend of emotions at play. Delving deeper to discern the underlying feelings can aid in better managing not only our anger but also behaviour and other emotions. Emotions like sadness, disappointment, loneliness, overwhelm, embarrassment, hurt, helpless, pain, frustrated, insecurity, hunger, grief, anxiety, stress, threatened, tired, contempt, guilt, jealousy, rejection, abandonment, scared, fear and shame.

Constructive anger involves expressing oneself in a manner that fosters reconciliation instead of retaliation (we will explore this more in the next chapter on conflict resolution). Recognising anger as an emotion, neither inherently right nor wrong, is crucial. Anger serves as a signal that something is amiss, stemming from a perception of a situation impacting someone or something we value.

Described as a reaction of indignation, anger is often a secondary emotion, masking underlying feelings of fear, hurt, and sadness. These emotions trigger a fight or flight response, prompting us to protect ourselves by confronting or withdrawing from a situation.

Various factors, including individuals, locations, or circumstances, can serve as triggers for anger. It is crucial to be mindful of anger, as while it is a natural and sometimes healthy emotion, excessive anger can result in adverse consequences. These can include heightened stress levels and physical health conditions.

John Ashfield (2010) states that regular or extended periods of anger are linked to conditions like depression, anxiety, and insomnia, as well as a variety of physical health issues such as elevated blood pressure, weakened immune system, ulcers, irritable bowel syndrome, heart disease and stroke.

Asserting that anger is a choice emphasises our control over its expression,

between healthy and unhealthy anger expression is essential. Healthy anger is communicated openly and clearly, allowing for resolution – while unhealthy anger manifests as rage, resentment, or passive-aggressive behaviours.

Encouraging the management of anger through patience, deep breaths, and activities like exercise or creative expression helps regulate emotional arousal. Reminding oneself that challenges are a part of life and that getting angry won't solve everything is a valuable perspective.

Acknowledging that anger is inherent in life's frustrations, pain, losses, and others' unpredictable actions, the focus shifts to adapting our response to these inevitable events.

Some of the Benefits of Managing Anger:

- **Energy for Achievement:** using the energy that anger generates in a positive way can propel you to achieve more than you thought possible (for example: fuel for my gym competition which I won 2nd place in a triatholon).
- **Choice of Response:** what you do with your anger matters. You have the power to choose constructive actions that can lead to improvement.
- **Acceptance of Anger:** it is okay to feel anger, especially if someone has wronged you. Acknowledging your emotions is the first step to managing them.

"Do not let the sun go down on your anger." (Ephesians 4:26)

Impact of Anger on our Brain and Body

The impact of anger on our brain and body begins with the initial spark, activating the amygdala. Anger may stem from emotions such as rejection or frustration, triggering the amygdala 'to turn on' which initiates the same stress response system in your brain and body. This system, involving the hypothalamus, pituitary gland, and adrenal glands, setting off a hormonal chain reaction, preparing your body to cope with the stress associated with anger.

The sequence unfolds as follows: the amygdala communicates with the hypothalamus, prompting the release of a CRH hormone. This hormone signals the pituitary gland, to release yet another hormone ACTH.

This hormone communicates with the adrenal glands, leading to the secretion of stress hormones like cortisol, adrenaline, and noradrenaline. As these hormones are produced, they swiftly affect your neurons and cells. Notably, this impact can often be unhelpful.

The alteration of your brain by stress hormones is a significant concern. An increase in cortisol levels can result in neurons absorbing excessive calcium through their membranes. This poses a problem as it may lead to overactive firing of cells and eventual cell death. Elevated cortisol levels can also contribute to the loss of neurons in the prefrontal cortex and hippocampus.

Diminished activity in the prefrontal cortex may hinder your ability to exercise sound judgment, preventing you from making good decisions or planning effectively for the future, particularly during moments of distress. Excessive cortisol in the hippocampus can further exacerbate the issue by causing neuron loss and impeding the formation of new ones. Consequently, this weakens short-term memory and obstructs the creation of new memories, making it difficult to recall information during arguments, for example.

Moreover, an excess of cortisol can lead to a decrease in serotonin, the hormone associated with happiness. The reduction in serotonin levels may intensify feelings of anger and physical pain, potentially contributing to more aggressive behaviour or feelings of depression. Clearly, these hormones wield a profound impact on the functioning of your body.

Anger triggers the release of stress hormones such as cortisol, adrenaline, and noradrenaline, providing a burst of energy to cope with challenging situations. While this response is beneficial in moderation, an excess or repeated exposure to these hormones can have adverse effects on vital bodily functions.

These effects include a slowing metabolism, reduced blood flow and digestive system function, compromised thyroid function, sensations of dry mouth, vision issues like tunnel vision or blurred vision, heightened sensitivity to light, increased pressure inside the eyes, more frequent headaches and migraines, elevated heart rate, blood pressure, blood glucose level, and blood fatty acid level. There is also an increased likelihood of stroke and heart attack, lowered bone density, a higher incidence of cancer and a greater susceptibility to viral infections.

Even after the feeling of anger subsides, the lingering impact on the body persists for an extended period. Additionally, the more frequently anger is experienced, the more these hormones continue to exert their effects.

Some Common Objections to Anger Management I Hear:

"Feeling angry is bad, and I shouldn't let myself get angry."

My response: feeling anger is a natural emotion, and it is not inherently bad. It is how we choose to respond to anger, that matters. You have the power to use anger constructively or not.

"I can't control my anger; it just takes over."

My response: while anger can be intense, you can learn techniques to manage and control your response. You have the ability to choose a constructive reaction.

"Being angry intimidates others and protects me."

My response: anger is a powerful emotion, it can protect you when you need it, however excess or repeated exposure to these hormones can have adverse effects on vital bodily functions, your mental health, physical pain levels and reducing your overall wellbeing.

Different Ways to Manage your Anger:

Anger is an emotion that can make you feel charged up, leading to impulsive actions. When angry, the brain may suggest that giving in to anger will bring relief. But as we have just read there is a cost, and the consequences can often be painful and detrimental. Expressing anger through venting or physical aggression might provide momentary satisfaction, but it can harm relationships and worsen situations over time.

- **Response-ability:** your ability to choose your response, Viktor Frankl (1963) conceived the term. In *Man's Search for Meaning*, a book written by Frankl, he said the only thing that cannot be taken away from someone is their freedom *"to choose one's attitude in any given set of circumstances, to choose one's own way"* human liberty, independence of mind and *"spiritual freedom in regard to behaviour and reaction to any given surroundings."* (1963, p 104). His surroundings were inside a concentration camp during WWII.

- **Forgiveness:** whilst this may not be a popular strategy for everyone it is still useful to ponder over – is the anger you hold onto healthy for YOU?

  Recognising the detrimental effects of holding onto destructive anger, including resentment and bitterness, suggests the importance of forgiveness. Forgiveness becomes a necessary step in releasing anger's grip over YOU and preventing ongoing damage.

  Choosing not to forgive means holding onto anger, with the other party often unaware of the impact on us. Forgiveness entails refraining from seeking revenge, liberating us from the stressful and damaging feelings associated with anger and resentment. Again, it comes down to YOUR personal choice.

- **Traffic Light:** I use the traffic light model when working with children. Picture your anger as a traffic light: 'Stop' to recognise it, 'Think' to understand where it comes from and decide how best to respond, and 'Go' with a positive action to address the anger (which will likely involve the assertiveness communication in *Chapter 1*).

- **Shifting Perspective:** anger can lead us to interpret non-verbal cues negatively. For instance, a smile from a co-worker might be perceived as sarcastic or aggressive. Pay more attention to the eyes of a person rather than their mouth to interpret emotions accurately, reducing reactivity and anger.

- **Practicing Mindfulness:** mindfulness involves staying present and aware of your thoughts and feelings without judgment. This practice can help you observe and manage anger more effectively. Mindfulness serves not only to diminish anger but also to alleviate anxiety and enhance our rational decision-making. By concentrating on the present moment, we can eliminate negative emotions from our decision-making process, allowing for more sensible choices.

  As mentioned earlier, anger often leads to recklessness and irrational thinking. Therefore, mindfulness assists in maintaining focus and promoting clear thinking before taking action. Engaging in mindfulness involves directing attention to bodily sensations, including breathing, physical feelings, and posture. Additionally, being attuned to our emotional state is another way to practice mindfulness.

- **Progressive Muscle Relaxation (PMR):** we used progressive muscle relaxation in the previous chapters, and it can equally help with anger management. A well-established relaxation technique known for its proven effectiveness in alleviating muscle tension and countering the 'fight or flight' anxiety response is progressive muscle relaxation. This method entails systematically tensing and then releasing muscles, allowing individuals to experience, and become aware of the sensation of tension. Whilst the technique is the same the wording of the script can be varied. See below for an alternate script and audio.

- The key principles of this approach involve sequentially tensing specific muscle groups to notice tension and subsequently relaxing the muscles, experiencing the gradual release of tension out of the body.

Example of a different PMR Script:

- Prepare yourself in a serene environment. Silence your phone and lower the lights. This is your moment, dedicated to absolute relaxation. Whether you choose to sit or lie down, ensure you're comfortably warm. Allow your hands to rest loosely in your lap or by your side. Now, gently close your eyes. Tune into your breath, observing the rise and fall of your abdomen with each inhalation and exhalation.
- Take a slow, deep breath in through your nose, filling your lungs completely. Now exhale through your mouth, letting the breath carry away any stress or tension. Another deep breath in, and a slow exhale, releasing any remaining tension. One more deep breath in, and let it go. Feel the subtle changes in your body, sensing the relaxation setting in.
- Let your breathing return to its natural rhythm. During this relaxation journey, I'll guide you to gently tense and then release various muscle groups. Please do this without straining, and if at any point you feel discomfort, simply relax, and breathe normally.
- Begin by focusing on your feet and toes. Inhale deeply through your nose, gradually curling your toes down, tensing the muscles in the soles of your feet. Hold briefly, and as you exhale, release the tension. Notice the sensation of relaxation flowing through your feet. Repeat this process, breathing in as you tense and exhaling as you release.
- Move your attention to your lower legs and calf muscles. Inhale deeply,

you exhale, let the tension dissolve. Once more, inhale, tighten your calf muscles, and exhale, releasing all tension.

- If you're lying down, straighten your legs to engage the muscles in the front of your thighs. If seated, push your heels down into the floor. Inhale deeply, tense your thigh muscles, hold briefly, and exhale, allowing the muscles to relax completely.
- Continue this process, gradually working your way up your body, tensing and releasing muscles in your buttocks, stomach, back, shoulders, and neck. With each breath, feel the tension melting away, leaving you in a state of deep relaxation.
- Shift your focus to your upper arms, forearms, hands, and fingers. Inhale deeply as you tighten each muscle group, holding briefly, and exhale as you release, enjoying the soothing sensation of relaxation.
- Finally, bring attention to your facial muscles. Inhale, squeezing your eyes shut and clenching your lips together. Hold briefly, and as you exhale, allow your facial muscles to relax. Open your mouth wide on an inhale, feeling the stretch in your jaw, and exhale, letting your mouth gently close.

Now, revel in the profound sense of relaxation that envelops your entire body. Take a few moments to rest, listen to the rhythm of your breath, and savour the warmth of physical tranquillity. If time allows, feel free to drift into a peaceful sleep, knowing you should awaken rejuvenated and fully relaxed.

✸ **Access to this recording:**
https://www.atfullpotential.com.au/the-challenge-journal

As I say to my sons, *"You are old enough and responsible now to make your own decisions, however you will also be accountable for their consequences."*

How do you express your anger?

....

Blow up, take it out on others, hold it in, be angry at yourself, seek revenge, hurt the person that hurt you?

What are helpful ways to express your anger?

....

Sometimes I like to write or journal, some people have written songs in order to express their pain and anger. Others hide away to protect the world from their responses. Some people play the drums; some people run, and others exercise (I prevailed in a mini- triatholon once largely driven by anger).

Summary

In this chapter, we examined the importance of managing anger, acknowledging it as a universal emotion with neither a right nor wrong aspect. Constructive anger involves recognising it as a **signal**, often masking underlying feelings. Various triggers can incite anger, requiring awareness to prevent **adverse** consequences such as stress-related health issues.

Behaviours in response to anger are portrayed as a **choice**, urging the distinction between healthy and unhealthy expressions. Techniques for anger management include deep breathing and activities like exercise or creative expression. The chapter highlights the benefits of managing anger, such as channelling energy for achievement and making thoughtful choices in responses.

The impact of anger on the brain and body is explored, emphasising the role of

by suggesting mindfulness and progressive muscle relaxation as a valuable technique for alleviating muscle tension and promoting relaxation.

Three Actions to Take:

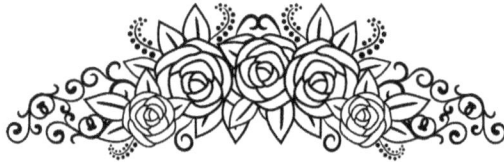

1. **Take a mindful approach** to understanding your underlying emotions, this can help manage anger. Circle the emotions that anger may have been a response to: sad, disappointed, lonely, overwhelmed, embarrassed, hurt, helpless, pain, frustrated, insecure, hungry, grief, anxiety, stress, threatened, tired, contempt, guilt, jealousy, rejection, abandonment, scared, fear and shame. Or write your own emotion if not listed here.

2. **Identify how you typically express your anger** and explore healthier ways to channel it.

3. **Consider engaging in a physical activity** to release anger and maintain emotional well-being. For example, swimming, kickboxing, cycling, jogging/walking. Alternatively use progressive muscle relaxation or mindfulness.

Remember that you have the ability to choose your response. It is your response-ability so try to choose a way that supports you.

Additional Information and Resources:

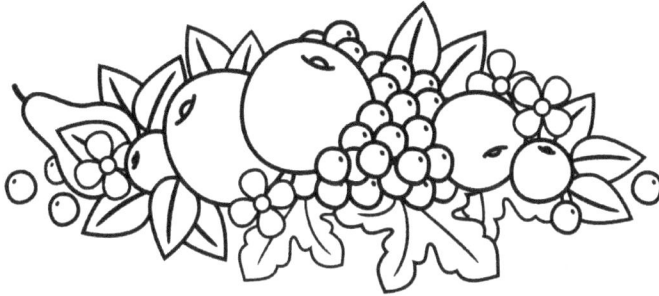

In the next chapter on conflict resolution, we will delve deeper into practical exercises and techniques to help you manage your anger effectively. If your anger significantly impacts your daily life and relationships, consider seeking guidance from a qualified therapist or counsellor with expertise in anger management.

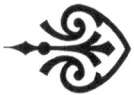

Safety Warning: If your anger or anger of another is putting you or others in danger, please seek professional help and keep as safe as possible. *(Please see the Help Organisations section at the end of this book for more information.)*

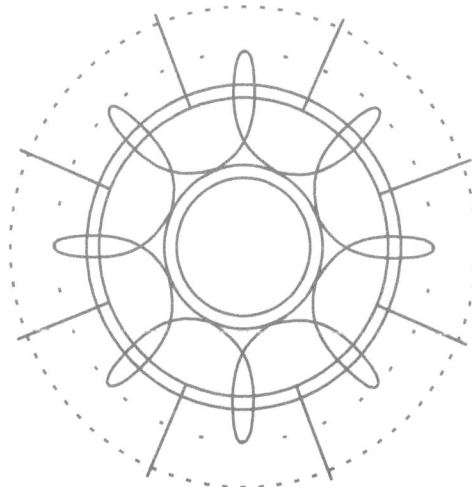

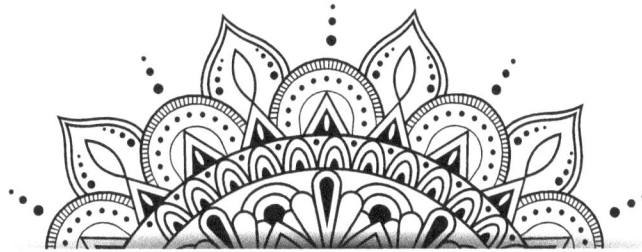

CHAPTER 11

Resolve Your Conflict

"Anger, fear, aggression. The dark side are they." (Yoda)

People often experience situations differently because they have unique thoughts, feelings, and experiences. In this chapter, we will explore steps to help resolve conflicts with respect and care for those involved. The benefits of using this approach to resolve conflicts are:

- **Respectful resolution:** this approach offers a respectful way to resolve conflicts, ensuring that all parties are heard.
- **New solutions:** this method provides an opportunity to come up with innovative solutions that both sides may not have initially considered, resulting in a win-win situation.
- **Mutual success:** both parties have the potential to experience a 'win,' whether through compromise or finding a mutually satisfying resolution. This is through an abundance framework.

- **Breaking the argument cycle:** by following these steps, you can prevent conflicts from escalating into prolonged arguments.
- **Incorporating past learning:** the conflict resolution steps incorporate lessons from previous chapters, communication, problem-solving and anger management, for example.

Abundance Model

Abundance is the opposite of scarcity.

Instead of coming from a finite frame of mind where if one person wins the other person must lose, this conflict resolution model allows for infinite ideas to resolve the conflict and come up with new solutions that may not have been apparent at first from a single individual perspective.

The contrast lies in the shift from a finite frame of mind where one person wins at the expense of the other to a model that promotes infinite ideas for conflict resolution, fostering new and creative solutions.

Stephen Covey (2004) in his book *The 7 Habits of Highly Effectual People* speaks about habit 4: Think WIN-WIN – not compromise but a better solution.

"Win-win is a belief in the Third Alternative. It's not your way or my way; it's a better way, a higher way." (Stephen R. Covey)

The Gottman Method and Relationships

When considering conflict within a relationship, it is crucial to determine whether a particular issue is **resolvable** or **perpetual**. Over half of relationship conflicts falls into the category of perpetual problems, which all couples inevitably encounter. These issues stem from the fundamental differences inherent in any two individuals, manifesting either as recurring clashes in personalities or disparities in lifestyle needs. Perpetual problems, which refers to recurring issues in a relationship that are often grounded in fundamental differences in personalities or lifestyle needs.

In the Gottman approach, perpetual problems are issues that couples will likely face repeatedly throughout their relationship. These problems arise from inherent differences between partners that are unlikely to be fully resolved. Examples could include differences in values, personality traits, or long-standing habits.

The Gottman Method emphasises that it is natural for couples to have perpetual problems, and the goal is not necessarily to eliminate these problems but to **manage** them effectively. The approach encourages couples to develop healthy communication skills, emotional intelligence, and a strong foundation of friendship to navigate these perpetual issues.

Rather than trying to 'solve' these problems, the focus is on creating understanding, acceptance, and **constructive dialogue** around them. Instead of seeking solutions for perpetual problems, the key lies in a couple's ability to establish an open dialogue about them.

Resolvable problems pertain to issues like housecleaning, child discipline, or in-law relationships. What might be a resolvable problem for one couple could be a

problem is **situational**, with the conflict revolving around a specific topic, often lacking deeper meaning. Solutions can be identified and maintained. However, unlike resolvable problems, perpetual problems persistently resurface, becoming recurring points of contention.

The Gottman Model prioritises building emotional intelligence and developing conflict management skills to enhance friendship within couples, fostering a shared meaning in their relationship.

The emphasis is not on solving perpetual problems but more in the way they are discussed. The goal is to establish a dialogue about perpetual problems that communicates acceptance of one's partner with humour, affection, and respect, actively managing unresolvable issues rather than allowing them to reach gridlock. Gridlocked discussions often result in painful exchanges or icy silence, frequently involving the Four Horsemen (criticism, contempt, stonewalling and defensiveness). (Gottman & Gottman, 2017)

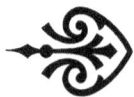

Safety Warning: If you believe that entering a conflict resolution situation may not be safe in your specific circumstances, such as in cases of domestic violence, or narcissistic relationships, it is crucial to seek professional advice before attempting. It may be an option to investigate mediation services to help you navigate this space safely. *(Please see the Help Organisations section at the end of this book for more information)*

Some objections and responses to learning conflict resolution skills:

"I have tried to resolve the conflict, but nothing has worked."

My response: you have been practising new techniques like communication, problem-solving and anger management which have been incorporated here. Practicing these techniques equips you with the skills to navigate the conflict resolution steps more effectively. Understanding these chapters gives you the best chance for successful resolution - especially when both parties respect and care for each other.

"It's too much effort."

My response: the effort you put into resolving the conflict is a choice. Consider whether the pain of the conflict is greater than the effort required to resolve it.

"Every time we try to discuss it, we get too angry, so it's better to avoid."

My response: learning how to manage anger can help create a conducive environment for fruitful discussions. Use what was learnt in *Chapter 10* on anger management which provides guidance for managing emotions during conflict resolution.

Consider the Gottman Method as it could be a perpetual problem. The first part of conflict resolution model can help. Even if the mutual solution is to respectfully agree to disagree.

"Fear is the path to the dark side...fear leads to anger...anger leads to hate...hates leads to suffering." (Yoda)

Ways to Resolve Conflict

Seeing different perspectives: understand that individuals may see situations differently due to their unique thoughts, feelings, and experiences. This is similar to the perpetual problems explained previously.

Seeing different perspectives is illustrated through visual examples below. Look at the first picture -do you see two people facing each other? Or do you see a goblet? Now look at the second picture – the goblet is easier to see simply because a border has framed the image, giving a different perspective.

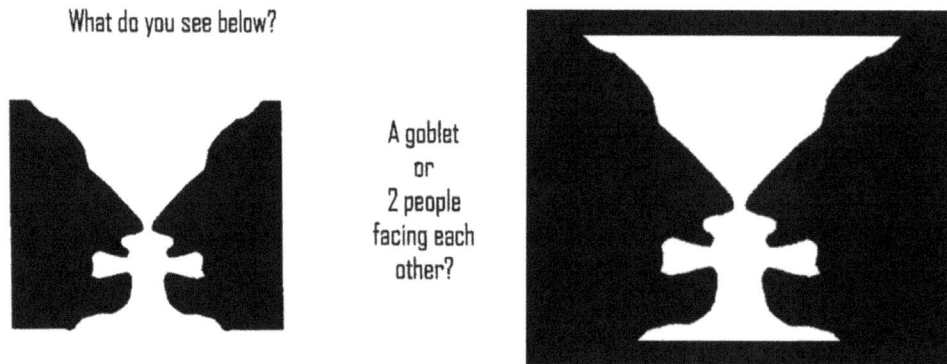

What do you see below?

A goblet
or
2 people
facing each
other?

(just by adding a border can help change the perspective)

Conflict Resolution Steps (see illustration): learn the eight conflict resolution steps, which involve active listening, assertive communication, problem-solving, and action planning to resolve conflicts. You may need a mediator to keep the conversation effective.

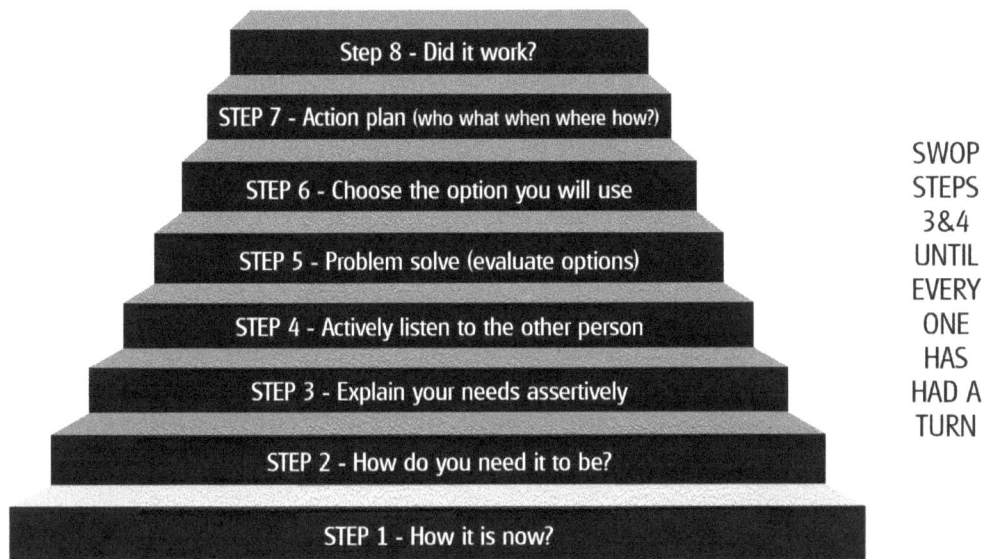

STEP
Step 8 - Did it work?
STEP 7 - Action plan (who what when where how?)
STEP 6 - Choose the option you will use
STEP 5 - Problem solve (evaluate options)
STEP 4 - Actively listen to the other person
STEP 3 - Explain your needs assertively
STEP 2 - How do you need it to be?
STEP 1 - How it is now?

SWOP STEPS 3&4 UNTIL EVERY ONE HAS HAD A TURN

CONFLICT RESOLUTION STEPS

Step 1 – Think about how the situation is now.

Step 2 – Think about how you want it to be.

Step 3 – Assertively express your needs (using I am... because... I need...) like we did in *Chapter 1*.

Step 4 – Listen to the other person (use reflective listening – listen to understand not to counterattack).

Repeat and swap Step 3 and 4.

Step 5 – Problem solve together (like we did in Chapter 3).

Step 6 – Choose the best option.

Step 7 – Action plan (**who** will do **what**, **when** and **how**).

Step 8 – Did it work? Check in with each other, is it resolved? If not go back to an earlier step and try again.

"Thousands of candles can be lighted from a single candle, and the life of the candle will not be shortened. Happiness never decreases by being shared." (Buddha)

Summary

This chapter discusses the varied nature of human experiences and how conflicts arise due to unique thoughts, feelings, and backgrounds. It emphasises a conflict resolution approach that promotes respect, new solutions, mutual success and breaking the argument cycle.

The abundance model is introduced as a shift from a finite mindset to one that fosters infinite ideas for resolution.

The Gottman Method is explored in the context of relationships, distinguishing between resolvable and perpetual problems. The focus is on managing perpetual issues through healthy communication, emotional intelligence, and friendship, rather than seeking complete solutions.

A diagram outlines ways to resolve conflict, including understanding different perspectives and the eight conflict resolution steps involving active listening, assertive communication, problem-solving and action planning. The steps include thinking about the current situation, expressing needs assertively, listening actively, problem-solving collaboratively, choosing the best option, creating an action plan, and checking in on resolution success.

Three Actions to Take:

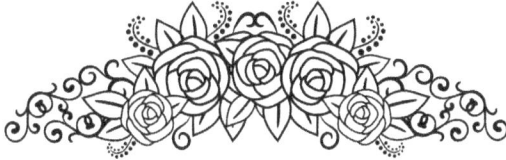

1. **Different perspectives (goblet illustration):** this concept emphasises that individuals may perceive situations differently based on their thoughts, feelings, and experiences. Is there a different perspective you could try to understand? If there is a constant conflict could it be a perpetual problem and not a resolvable problem? If this is the case, then constructive open dialogue is helpful.

2. **Conflict resolution steps (illustration):** use these eight steps to guide conflict resolution, facilitating effective communication, active listening, and problem-solving to reach a mutually beneficial solution.

3. **Moving forward:** good communicating involves reflective listening and aim to work toward a new solution that may not have been apparent before.

Additional Information and Resources:

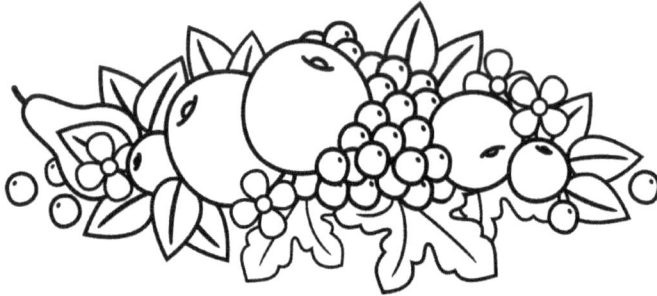

In the next chapter, after learning about communication, realistic thinking, problem solving, depression, goal setting, schemas, anxiety, mindfulness, stress management, anger management and conflict resolution, we will develop a relapse prevention plan.

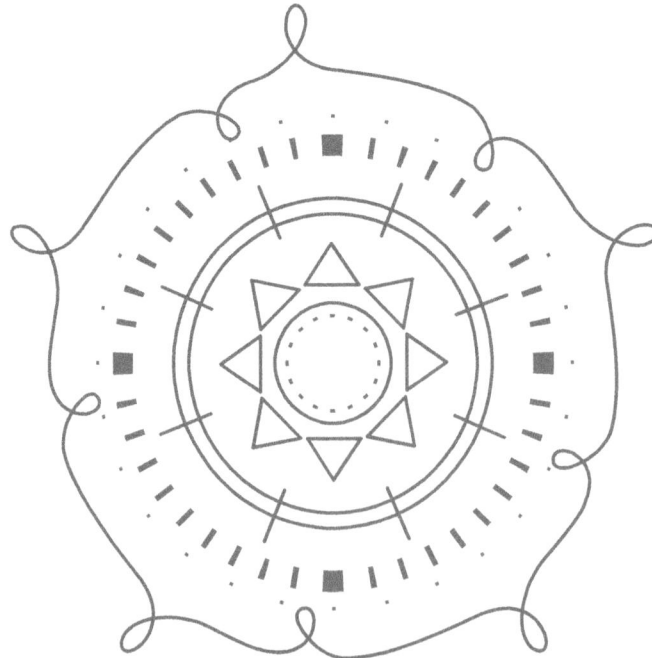

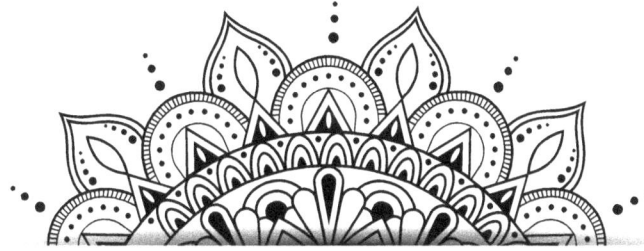

CHAPTER 12

Prevent Any Relapse

"Tell me and I forget. Teach me and I remember. Involve me and I learn."
(Benjamin Franklin)

Relapse Prevention is about recognising early warning signs indicative of mental ill-health and proactively implementing safety plans to prevent subsequent relapses and minimise its impact. The benefits of relapse prevention is:

- **Identification of warning signs:** recognising and documenting early warning signs indicative of declining mental health is a crucial part of relapse prevention.
- **Early intervention:** early detection of these signs increases the chances of preventing a relapse from occurring or at least minimising the impact.
- **Minimising mental health decline:** the earlier you identify the signs and seek help the less chance your mental health can deteriorate.
- **Support from loved ones:** sharing your relapse prevention plan with

to recognise signs of deteriorating mental health particularly when you might not be in the right mindset.
- **Proactive action:** creating an action plan and communicating it to others is a proactive approach to mental health maintenance.

> *"Our greatest glory is not in never falling,*
> *but in rising every time we fall."*
> (Confucius)

Early warning signs encompass changes in **thoughts, feelings** and **behaviours** that indicate a decline in your mental health. They can be common or unique to each individual.

Action Plan

This is a set of actions to be taken if you notice the warning signs of relapse. It includes steps to prevent further deterioration in your mental health.

Examples of resistance often heard regarding relapse prevention plans and my responses:

"Why do I need a relapse prevention plan?"

My response: the importance of identifying early warning signs and documenting them can significantly aid in preventing relapses. Having a plan in place allows you to take action in case things worsen, ultimately minimising the impact on your mental health.

"Why should others be involved in my relapse prevention?"

My response: sharing your relapse prevention plan with others is crucial because sometimes you may not be the best judge of your own warning signs. In times when your mental health is deteriorating, having a support network that understands and follows the plan can make a significant difference.

Preventing relapse is a plan to notice the warning signs early and act.

The warning signs are changes in behaviours, thoughts and feelings that are present when a person's mental health is declining. They are a change in the normal behaviours, thoughts, and feelings that the person has. There are several common changes in behaviours, thoughts, and feelings that many people experience when their mental health is declining.

Example:

Thoughts: more negative like 'I cannot cope' when usually the thoughts are more realistic or neutral.
Feelings: depressed, unmotivated, and overwhelmed.
Behaviour: avoiding social occasions when they are usually quite social.

However, there can also be unique behaviours, thoughts and feelings that only occur when that unique person's mental health is declining. This is why it is important to create a personalised relapse prevention plan for each person and not just use a generic relapse prevention plan that may miss characteristic signs.

Example:

Thoughts: 'the world would be better off without me', when usually they are optimistic.
Feelings: teary for no reason, unusually more emotional.
Behaviour: start drinking through the week when previously they didn't drink very much at all, except for social occasions.

It is beneficial to have those around us know what the relapse prevention plan is.

This list of early warning behaviours, thoughts, and feelings is suggested to be identified and communicated to trusted friends, family, doctors, and therapists because sometimes we are not the best judge of these warning signs.

We may not notice the decline ourselves due to the current state of our mental health.

Our family and friends may notice changes exhibited quicker than we do.

How to Do the Relapse Prevention Plan

Identify the **early warning signs** and list them:

- Identify the **thoughts** that are more likely to occur when your mental health is declining e.g., thinking to oneself, *"I am not good enough, I will never be good enough."*

- Identify the **feelings** that are more likely to occur when your mental health is declining e.g., feeling unmotivated because there is no point even trying.

- Identify the **behaviours** that are more likely to occur when your mental health is declining e.g., taking less care with personal hygiene.

Action Plan:

Write down what actions you will take if these symptoms occur.

For example: make appointment to see my doctor, see my specialist, pick up my pharmacy script, phone my friend, list strategies that have worked for me in the past, take up writing in this journal again.

To prevent relapses, you need to be able to identify your early warning signs.

Signs

List some of the thoughts you have when your mental health is not at its best:

Thoughts

....

....

List some of the feelings you have when your mental health is not at its best:

Feelings

....

....

....

List some of the behaviours you have when your mental health is not at its best:

Behaviour

....

....

....

Once the warning signs are documented, you can communicate it to others and include an action plan for what you need to do to prevent further relapse. What needs to happen goes into the action plan.

For Example:

Include doctors name and telephone number so prompt appointment can be made, when it is mental health related, communicate that when booking the

Have the relapse prevention sheet with the thoughts, feelings and behaviours listed. You can use this book to list the plan.

List any medications and dosage; previous medication; has there been a change to your medication recently?

List psychologist/psychiatrist/paediatrician and contact number(s).

Action Plan

e.g., contact local GP and book appointment (ask someone to book for me if I cannot)

....

....

....

If suicidal plans are present, then attend hospital emergency department or call an ambulance.

Closest hospital name and address:

....

....

Relapse Prevention

Share this with a trusted person when you're ready.

Early warning signs that may indicate that my mental health is declining:

Thoughts

- ❑
- ❑
- ❑
- ❑

Feelings

- ❑
- ❑
- ❑
- ❑

Behaviours

- ❑
- ❑
- ❑

Action

When I notice these symptoms, I can utilise one or more of the strategies I have found helpful in the past. These may include for example:

❏ Book appointment with GP
❏ Book appointment with therapist
❏ Speak to my trusted person
❏ Check medications and dosages (any recent changes)
❏
❏

GP Name and Number ....
Therapist Name and Number ....
Local Hospital Name and Number ....
Help organisations ....

"Know all the theories, master all the techniques, but as you touch a human soul be just another human soul." (C.G. Jung)

Summary

Relapse Prevention is about recognising early warning signs of deteriorating mental health and proactively implementing safety plans. Early Intervention involves the timely identification of signs, and appropriate execution of safety plans, increasing the likelihood of preventing a relapse or minimising its impact.

Three Actions to Take:

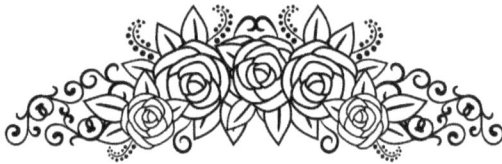

1. **Identify your warning signs in the relapse prevention plan provided:** recognise behaviours, thoughts, and feelings that are more likely to occur when your mental health is declining. For example, changes in personal hygiene, self-doubting thoughts, and feelings of demotivation. Take time to identify the early warning signs specific to your mental health.

2. **Create an action plan:** write down the actions you will take if these symptoms occur. For instance, scheduling an appointment with your doctor. Develop a personalised action plan for you to follow if the warning signs appear.

3. **Share your plan by taking a photo:** communicate your relapse prevention plan with trusted friends, family, doctors, and therapists to ensure you have support when you might not notice the signs yourself.

Additional Information and Resources:

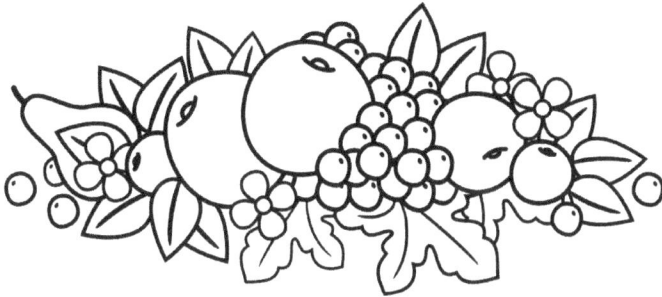

Congratulations, you have reached the end of this journey!

You have learned about valuable tools and insights to help maintain your mental wellness and achieve a healthier, happier life.

Revisit this book whenever you need to refresh your memory and journal.

I wish you well and may the force be with you.

Katrina x

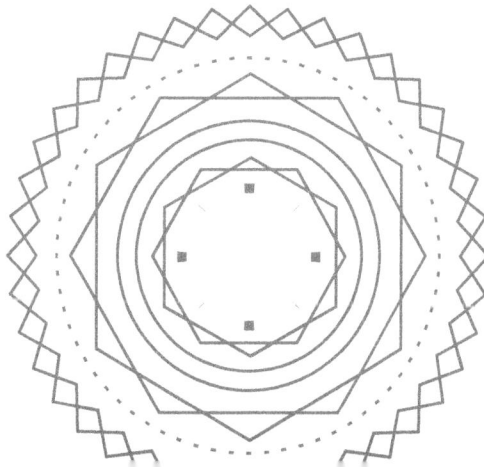

Afterword

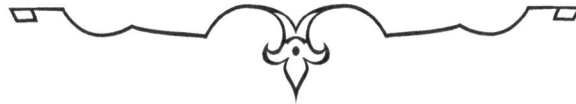

The Evolution of The Challenge Journal Over the Years

Since *The Challenge Journal's* First Edition (2005) and Second Edition (2011) that were self-published, significant advancements in psychology and the world in general have taken place.

This Third Edition includes some of those important improvements, keeping pace with the ever-growing landscape of knowledge and understanding. I am also dedicated to extending the inclusive intent of this book from its inception, striving to make it as accessible as possible to a diverse audience of readers and listeners.

Inclusivity is a powerful lens through which to view the world and share insights. It's like inviting more voices to the table, enriching the conversation, and making sure that the wisdom within the pages resonates with a diverse audience. Building that bridge to many readers and listeners, creating a space where a wide range of perspectives can find value and connection.

This Third Edition will be expanded onto several different platforms to enhance inclusivity. By diversifying the ways in which this content is presented – audibly for example – it essentially casts a wider net to capture various audience preferences

About the Author

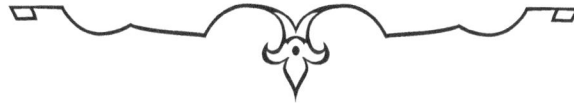

Katrina Langhorn is a registered psychologist, qualified teacher, and business coach.

For over 20 years, Katrina has worked in private practice helping thousands of patients. During that time, Katrina has also worked across many different settings including schools, hospitals, and correctional facilities.

Katrina has worked with several organisations including *Youth off the Streets* and *Disability Services Australia*. Katrina has also volunteered for *LIFELINE's* 24-hour crisis support and suicide prevention hotline. Katrina mentors and supervises provisional psychology interns and university students.

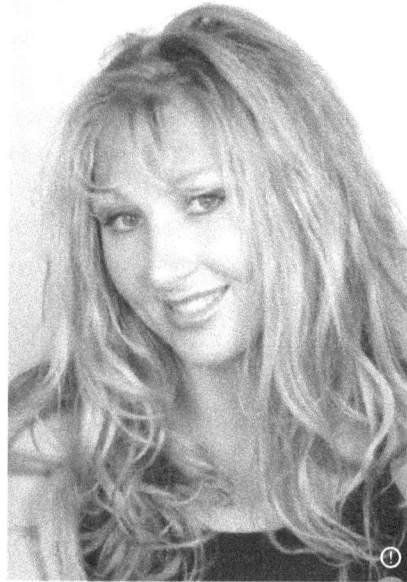

Today, Katrina travels across Australia, facilitating workshops and presenting strategies from *The Challenge Journal*. Katrina was invited to speak to the United Services Union, has been a regular facilitator for over a decade with Positive Partnerships and over the last few years for the *Business Bricks Empowerment*

References and Further Reading

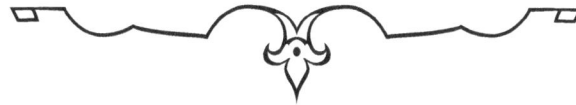

Abramson, L. Y., Seligman, M. E. P., & Teasdale, J. D. (1978). Learned helplessness in humans: Critique and reformulation. *Journal of Abnormal Psychology, 87,* 49-74.

Ackerman, C. (2018, March 24). *Learned Helplessness: Seligman's Theory of Depression (+ Cure).* PositivePsychology.com. https://positivepsychology.com/learned-helplessness-seligman-theory-depression-cure/

Adolescent Moral Development Lab. (2018). *Psychology of Purpose.* [Review of *Psychology of Purpose.*]. Claremont Graduate University for Prosocial Consulting and the John Templeton Foundation.

Anderson, N.B., Belar, C.D., Breckler, S.J., Nordal, K.C., Ballard, D.W., Bufka, L.F., Bossolo, L., Bethune, S., Brownawell, A., Wiggins, K. (2015). *Stress in America: Paying with Our Health.* [Review of *Stress in America: Paying with Our Health.*]. American Psychological Association.

Ashfield, J. (2010).Taking care of yourself and your family : a resource book for good mental health. Norwood, South. Australia: Peacock Publications for Beyondblue, the National Depression Initiative.

Australian Bureau of Statistics. (2020-2022). National Study of Mental Health and Wellbeing. ABS. https://www.abs.gov.au/statistics/health/mental-health/national-study-mental-health-and-wellbeing/2020-2022.

Australian Bureau of Statistics. (2023, October 5). Two in five Australians have experienced a mental disorder. ABS. https://www.abs.gov.au/media-centre/media-releases/two-five-australians-have-experienced-mental-disorder.

Australian Psychological Society. (2015). *Stress & wellbeing HOW AUSTRALIANS ARE COPING WITH LIFE.* https://psychology.org.au/getmedia/ae32e645-a4f0-4f7c-b3ce-dfd83237c281/stress-wellbeing-survey.pdf

Breckler, S. J., & Ballard, D. W. (2014). *Stress in America-Are Teens Adopting Adults' Stress Habits?* https://www.apa.org/news/press/releases/stress/2013/stress-report.pdf

Carretié, L., Mercado, F., Tapia, M., & Hinojosa, J. A. (2001). Emotion, attention, and the 'negativity bias,' studied through event-related potentials. *International Journal of Psychophysiology, 41*(1), 75–85.

Covey, S. R. (2004). *The 7 habits of highly effective people : restoring the character ethic* ([Rev. ed.]). Free Press.

Du, C., Zan, M. C. H., Cho, M. J., Fenton, J. I., Hsiao, P. Y., Hsiao, R., Keaver, L., Lai, C.-C., Lee, H., Ludy, M.-J., Shen, W., Swee, W. C. S., Thrivikraman, J., Tseng, K.-W., Tseng, W.-C., Doak, S., Folk, S. Y. L., & Tucker, R. M. (2021). The Effects of Sleep Quality and Resilience on Perceived Stress, Dietary Behaviors, and Alcohol Misuse: A Mediation-Moderation Analysis of Higher Education Students from Asia, Europe, and North America during the COVID-19 Pandemic. *Nutrients, 13*(2),

Epton, T., Currie, S., & Armitage, C. J. (2017). Unique effects of setting goals on behavior change: Systematic review and meta-analysis. *Journal of Consulting and Clinical Psychology*, *85*(12), 1182–1198. https://doi.org/10.1037/ccp0000260

Frankl, V. E. (2006). *Man's Search for Meaning*. Boston, MA: Beacon Press.

Gottman, J., Gottman, J. (2017) *Level 1 clinical training*. The Gottman institute.

Guidelines - Mindframe, mindframe.org.au (2023).

Hari, J. (2022). *Stolen Focus*. Crown Publishing Group (NY).

Hetrick, S., Parker, A., Bailey, A., Cahill, S., Rice. S., Garvin, T., Phelan, M., and Davey, C., (2015). *Cognitive–behavioural therapy for depression in young people: a treatment manual.* Melbourne: Orygen, The National Centre of Excellence in Youth Mental Health.

Lazarus, R.S. *Psychological Stress and the Coping Process*. McGraw-Hill; New York, NY, USA: 1966.

Lee-Knight, K., & Napier, C. (2018). From high performance to clinical practice. *British Journal of Sports Medicine*, *52*(24), 1541–1542. https://doi.org/10.1136/bjsports-2018-100307

Leow, S., Jackson, B., Alderson, J.A., Guelfi, K.J., Dimmock, J.A., (2018). A Role for Exercise in Attenuating Unhealthy Food Consumption in Response to Stress. *Nutrients*. 6;10(2):176.

MacDonald, W. (2003). The Impact of Job Demands and Workload on Stress and

Marx, W., Moseley, G., Berk, M., Jacka, F. Nutritional psychiatry: the present state of the evidence. *Proc Nutr Soc*. 2017 Nov;76(4):427-436.

Matthews, G. (2007). *The Impact of Commitment, Accountability, and Written Goals on Goal Achievement.* Psychology | Faculty Presentations, Department of Psychology, Dominican University of California.

Rejeski, W. J., Thompson, A., Brubaker, P. H., & Miller, H. S. (1992). Acute exercise: buffering psychosocial stress responses in women. *Health psychology: official journal of the Division of Health Psychology, American Psychological Association, 11*(6), 355–362. https://doi.org/10.1037//0278-6133.11.6.355

Richardson, B. (2022). Assertiveness Statistics & Facts: NEW Research For 2022. Acuity Training. https://www.acuitytraining.co.uk/news-tips/assertiveness-facts-research/

Salleh, M.R. Life event, stress and illness. *Malays J Med Sci.* 2008 Oct;15(4):9-18.

Selye, H. (1974). Stress without Distress. Philadelphia, PA: Lippincott pp. 26–39.

Siegel, D.J. (2010). *Mindsight: The New Science of Personal Transformation*. New York, NY: Bantam Books.

Vaish, A., Grossmann, T., & Woodward, A. (2008). Not all emotions are created equal: the negativity bias in social-emotional development. *Psychological Bulletin, 134*(3), 383–403.

Watson, N.F., Badr, M.S., Belenky. G., Bliwise. D.L., Buxton. O.M., Buysse. D., Dinges. D.F., Gangwisch. J., Grandner. M.A., Kushida. C., Malhotra. R.K., Martin. J.L., Patel. S.R., Quan. S.F., Tasali. E. Recommended Amount of Sleep for a Healthy

Adult: A Joint Consensus Statement of the American Academy of Sleep Medicine and Sleep Research Society. *Sleep*. 2015 Jun 1;38(6):843-4.

World Health Organization. (2023, September 27). *Anxiety disorders*. www.who.int; World Health Organization. https://www.who.int/news-room/fact-sheets/detail/anxiety-disorders

Wu, W. (2009, February 8). *Learned helplessness: How to tame a baby elephant.* [Personal Blog]. Retrieved from https://waynewu.wordpress.com/2009/02/08/learned-helplessness/

Yerkes, R.M., Dodson, J.D. (1908). The relation of strength of stimulus to rapidity of habit-formation. *Journal of Comparative Neurology and Psychology*. 18 (5): 459–482.

Young, J. E. (2007). *Schema Therapy*. American Psychological Assoc.

Australian and International Help Organisations

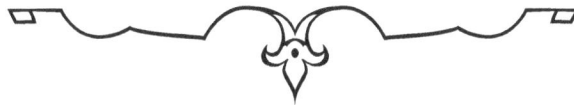

"Building a better tomorrow – behind every Veteran and Emergency Service First responder there is a human that has sacrificed through duty – thank you for your service."
(First Responders Support Hub)

Crisis Support Services:

24 hours, 7 days
Lifeline: 13 11 14
Suicide Call Back Service: 1300 659 467
Beyond Blue: 1300 224 636
MensLine Australia: 1300 789 978
Kids Helpline: 1800 551 800
13YARN: 13 92 76

First Responders Support Hub (Australia):

https://www.avconnect.org.au/first-responders-support

Information resources and links not only for the Australian Military Veterans and

Services, Police, Rescue services, State Emergency Service, Correctional, Surf lifesaving and Volunteer Marine Rescue.

Domestic Abuse:

If you are currently experiencing domestic abuse, for help in Australia, contact 1800RESPECT available 24 hours a day, 7 days a week on 1800737732.

Safe and Together Institute (International)

For international readers, please contact *Alliance for HOPE International* – focused on creating innovative, collaborative, trauma-informed, hope-centred approaches to meeting the needs of survivors of domestic violence, sexual assault, child abuse, elder abuse, and human trafficking.
https://safeandtogetherinstitute.com/international-domestic-violence-resources/

Relationships Australia:

1300364277
https://www.relationshipsnsw.org.au/support/services/
family-dispute-resolution-mediation/
International Mediation Institute

Reach-Out Australia Online:

https://au.reachout.com/mental-health-issues

Open Arms:

Veterans and families counselling 24 hr crisis support: 1800011046

Wounded Warrior Project for PTSD (America):

https://www.onceasoldier.org

Online CBT:

This Way Up, St Vincent's Hospital: www.thiswayup.org.au

Blackdog:

The Black Dog Institute is a not-for-profit organisation for diagnosis, treatment, and prevention of mood disorders such as depression, anxiety, and bipolar disorder.

www.blackdoginstitute.org.au

https://www.blackdoginstitute.org.au/wp-content/uploads/2020/04/19-dailymoodchart.pdf

My Local Emergency Department is: ....

Psychology Dictionary

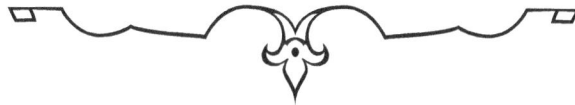

- **Acceptance and Commitment Therapy:** a therapeutic approach that emphasises accepting difficult thoughts and feelings, being mindful of the present moment and committing to actions aligned with personal values. It seeks to enhance psychological flexibility by fostering acceptance, mindfulness, and commitment to positive behaviour change.
- **Affective disorders:** or mood disorders, involve disruptions in mood regulation, leading to persistent changes in emotions. Examples include major depressive disorder and bipolar disorder, impacting daily life and often requiring treatment such as therapy or medication.
- **Automatic Thoughts:** quick, spontaneous, and often subconscious cognitions that occur in response to situations, influencing emotions and behaviours.
- **Behavioural Activation:** a therapeutic approach that focuses on encouraging individuals to engage in positive, rewarding activities to alleviate symptoms of depression or other mental health challenges.
- **Bipolar Disorder:** involves alternating depressive episodes and manic symptoms, including mood shifts, increased activity, and risky behaviour. Effective treatments, such as psychoeducation, stress reduction and medication, exist to manage the condition and reduce the risk of suicide.
- **Characterological**: the characteristics or traits related to an individual's character, especially those that are enduring and define one's personality.

behaviour, attitudes, and overall demeanour over an extended period. In psychology and personality theory, characterological traits are often considered fundamental aspects of an individual's personality structure.

- **Cognitive Behavioural Interventions:** involves therapeutic approaches that target and modify dysfunctional thought patterns and behaviours to enhance mental health.
- **Cognitive Behavioural Therapy (CBT):** a goal-oriented therapeutic approach that addresses and modifies dysfunctional thought patterns and behaviours, aiming to promote positive changes in emotional wellbeing and overall mental health.
- **Cognitive Bias:** refers to systematic patterns of deviation from norm or rationality in judgment, often leading to perceptual distortion, illogical interpretation, or irrationality in decision-making.
- **Cognitive Dissonance:** the discomfort felt when holding conflicting beliefs or attitudes, prompting individuals to seek harmony by adjusting their thoughts or behaviours.
- **Cognitive Distortions:** irrational thought patterns that contribute to negative emotions and behaviour. They involve biased ways of interpreting information, often leading to a skewed perception of reality. Identifying and challenging these distortions is a key aspect of CBT.
- **Cognitive Restructuring:** a therapeutic method that involves identifying and changing negative thought patterns to promote more positive and balanced thinking.
- **Complex Post-Traumatic Stress Disorder (C-PTSD):** a psychological condition that can result from prolonged exposure to traumatic events, often involving prolonged interpersonal trauma, such as chronic abuse or captivity. It shares features with PTSD but includes additional symptoms like difficulties with emotional regulation, interpersonal relationships, and a distorted self-perception. C-PTSD is often associated with repeated,

- **Daily Diary:** a written record or journal where individuals document their daily experiences, activities, thoughts, and emotions. It serves as a tool for self-reflection, allowing individuals to track and analyse their daily life, identify patterns, and gain insights into their thoughts and behaviours over time.
- **Depression:** a mental health disorder characterised by persistent feelings of sadness, loss of interest or pleasure in activities, changes in appetite and sleep patterns, low energy and difficulty concentrating. It can negatively impact a person's daily life, functioning and overall wellbeing.
- **Distraction:** techniques that involve shifting attention away from distressing thoughts or emotions by engaging in alternative, positive activities to provide temporary relief.
- **Emotional Reasoning:** where an individual relies on their emotions as the primary basis for forming conclusions, making decisions, or interpreting situations, rather than relying on objective evidence or logical reasoning. This can lead to subjective and potentially irrational judgments and behaviours.
- **Eustress:** a term used to describe positive or beneficial stress. Unlike distress, which is negative and harmful, eustress refers to stress that can be motivating, exciting and can enhance one's performance or wellbeing. It's associated with positive experiences and challenges that, while demanding, contribute to personal growth and achievement.
- **General Adaptation Syndrome (GAS):** a three-stage model describing the body's response to stress: alarm, resistance, and exhaustion. It highlights how the body adapts to stressors but may suffer if stress persists.
- **Graded Exposure:** a therapeutic technique that involves gradual and systematic exposure to anxiety-inducing stimuli or situations. It is used to help individuals overcome fears and anxiety by incrementally facing and adapting to the feared stimuli in a controlled manner.
- **Guided Imagery:** a form of focused visualisation where individuals are

script. It often includes verbal cues and prompts to direct the person's imagination in a specific way.

- **Hierarchy Ladder:** a structured system where fear evoking situations are ranked using a SUDS fear rating from lowest to highest.
- **Hyperventilation:** is rapid and shallow breathing, taking in more air than the body needs. It can be caused by stress or anxiety, leading to symptoms like dizziness and tingling.
- **Interoception:** is the capacity to detect and recognise internal physiological sensations, encompassing an awareness of bodily functions like heart rate, breathing patterns, and digestive activity. In essence, interoception enables us to attune to the physical sensations emerging from within our bodies.
- **Learned Helplessness:** a phenomenon seen in humans and other animals when they've been conditioned to anticipate pain, suffering, or discomfort without any means of avoiding it. This behaviour is learned, shaped by experiences where the individual either genuinely lacks control over their circumstances or just believes they have no control.
- **Mental Flow:** a state of focused and immersive engagement in a mental or cognitive activity, characterised by deep concentration, heightened awareness and a sense of enjoyment or fulfillment.
- **Metacognition:** the awareness and understanding of one's own thinking.
- **Microexpressions:** fast involuntary facial expressions that expose true emotion.
- **Mindfulness:** the intentional and non-judgmental awareness of the present moment, encompassing thoughts, feelings, bodily sensations, and surrounding environment.
- **Motivational Interviewing:** a counselling technique to elicit behavioural change by helping clients explore their own ambivalence.
- **Narrative Therapy:** sees individuals as storytellers of their own lives. It separates people from problems, challenges negative narratives and

non-pathologizing and aims to empower individuals by reshaping their narratives for positive change.

- **Negative Bias:** refers to the tendency of the human mind to give more importance and attention to negative information or experiences compared to positive ones. It influences perceptions, memories and decision-making, often leading individuals to focus on and remember adverse events more strongly than positive ones.

- **Outcome Probability Bias:** the tendency to overestimate the likelihood of a feared outcome occurring.

- **Post-Traumatic Stress Disorder (PTSD):** a mental health condition that can develop in individuals who have experienced or witnessed a traumatic event. Symptoms may include flashbacks, nightmares, severe anxiety, and uncontrollable thoughts about the event, persisting beyond the initial trauma.

- **Progressive Muscle Relaxation (PMR):** a relaxation technique involving the systematic tensing and relaxing of muscle groups to reduce overall stress and promote relaxation.

- **Psychoeducation:** is an approach that educates individuals and their families about mental health conditions, treatments, and coping strategies to enhance understanding and self-management.

- **Readiness to Change Graph:** visually represents an individual's readiness for a specific change, plotting the importance of the change against confidence in making it. It helps assess mindset and guides strategies for personal development or goal setting.

- **Response Prevention (Exposure and Response Prevention – ERP):** a therapy technique that involves intentionally avoiding or disrupting habitual behaviours to break the link between a trigger and an undesired response.

- **Rumination:** repetitive negative thinking or dwelling on distress and their causes.

- **Schema:** in psychology, a schema is a mental framework formed

information, impacting how they perceive, remember, and understand new information.

- **Sleep Hygiene:** refers to a set of practices and habits that promote good quality sleep. It involves maintaining a consistent sleep schedule, creating a comfortable sleep environment, limiting stimulants like caffeine, establishing a bedtime routine, reducing screen time before bed, engaging in regular exercise, managing stress, and watching diet close to bedtime. Following these practices can contribute to better sleep quality and overall wellbeing.

- **Stages of Change:** is a model outlining the various phases individuals undergo when making behavioural changes. They typically include precontemplation, contemplation, preparation, action, maintenance, and sometimes relapse.

- **Suicidal Ideation:** refers to thoughts or contemplation of suicidal behaviours. It is a serious and concerning aspect of mental health that may indicate an individual is experiencing significant emotional distress.

- **Switch-Cost Effect:** is the slowdown in reaction time and efficiency when people shift between different mental tasks or activities.

- **Thought Cue Cards:** concise cards containing alternative, constructive thoughts and prompts designed to help individuals navigate and respond to challenging or anxiety-provoking situations.

- **Thought Monitoring Record:** a tool used in CBT to track and analyse thoughts in relation to specific situations, emotions, and behaviours. It helps individuals identify automatic thoughts and challenge them to find a more balanced thought.

- **Thought Stopping:** a CBT technique where individuals interrupt and disrupt negative thoughts by consciously saying 'stop' to themselves, often followed by replacing the negative thoughts with more positive or constructive ones.

- **Visualisation:** a mental technique where individuals create a mental image or scenario in their mind. It involves using the power of imagination to see, feel and experience something without the direct sensory input.
- **Waffle:** while not specifically a psychological word but in the essence of inclusive language and direct explicit teaching, this word means to speak at length in a vague manner.
- **Window of Tolerance:** the optimal range of emotional arousal where a person can effectively cope with stress. If arousal is too high or too low, it can lead to difficulties in managing emotions.
- **Worry Time:** a designated period set aside each day for focused contemplation of concerns or negative thoughts, helping manage and control worrying.

Further Testimonials

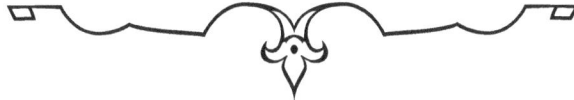

"This work is super helpful for everyone!"

Susan, Nutritionist, The Way to Health

"The Challenge Journal is packed with practical wisdom and actionable advice. It's a roadmap to self-discovery and positive transformation. Highly recommend for anyone seeking genuine, lasting change in their life."

Dianne, Director, EmpowerU

"What an amazing tool for navigating all sorts of relationships: personal and business. These steps are simple to follow and will help change the way we face challenging situations."

Tia, Tia Veech Everyday Solutions

"Excited to read and learn more on ways to enhance my thinking. It's definitely a challenge to try and improve certain habits that have created over the years. Such a great read!"

Sharon, Beautician, Exotic Skin Co

"It's written from the heart and has very practical tips that you can use immediately. It's not just a 'tell' book, it's a resource that will definitely get used in my business and home."

"I find the book easy to read and set out in a format that anyone struggling can understand. I look forward to sharing this with the homeless people we work with."

Sharon, No Home, My Home Project

"Running a business can be highly stressful, with challenges such as financial pressure, competition, workforce management, and maintaining a healthy work-life balance. Maintaining good mental health helps business owners cope with stress, prevent burnout, build, and maintain healthy relationships both in the workplace and outside of the workplace, and foster resilience. The Challenge Journal provides business owners (and others) with the tools to improve their communication, solve problems and make sound decisions, increase their productivity, manage stress, and achieve goals while allowing the mental space for creativity and innovation. A healthy mind helps to create a healthy business."

**Debbie, Business Consultant,
Advisor and Coach, Debbie Roberts Consulting**

Bonus Offer

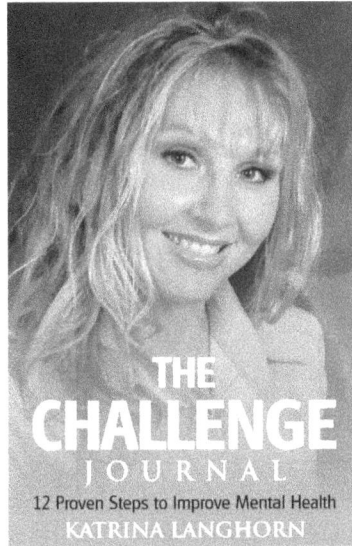

THE
CHALLENGE
JOURNAL
12 Proven Steps to Improve Mental Health
KATRINA LANGHORN

Offer 1: Would you like to print the illustrations, diagrams, and journaling in this book?

Download for free:

FREE giveaway
go to: https://www.atfullpotential.com.au

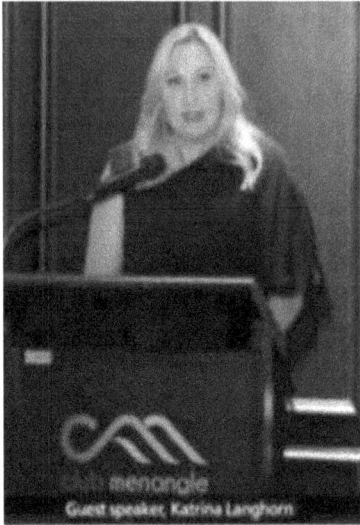
Guest speaker, Katrina Langhorn

Bonus Offer 2: Speaker Bio

To ensure a successful workshop or conference, having a facilitator who engages effectively with the audience, offering practical and achievable information and strategies, is crucial. It is essential that the content is grounded in scientific knowledge and presented in a way that is personally comprehensible for the success of the event.

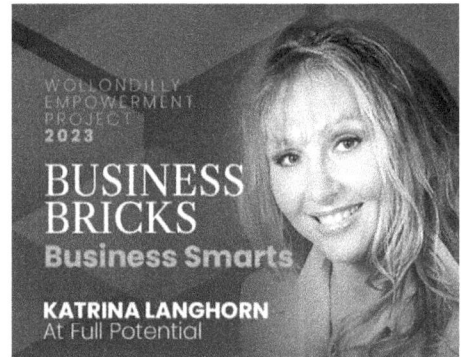

WOLLONDILLY EMPOWERMENT PROJECT 2023

BUSINESS BRICKS
Business Smarts

KATRINA LANGHORN
At Full Potential

Katrina Langhorn is an experienced conference and keynote speaker, lauded for her inviting and conversational approach. Her extensive professional background is firmly grounded in both academic knowledge with practical skills. Recognising that an exceptional presentation hinges on engaging delivery through stories and practical examples, Katrina ensures her audience takes home a meaningful message that fosters learning and personal growth.

With a career spanning over 20 years in the

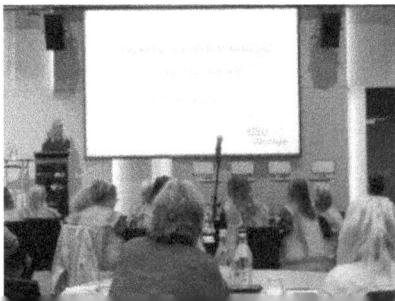

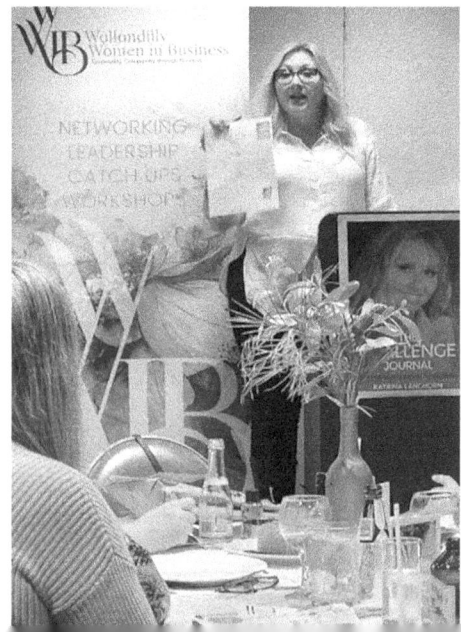

and education, Katrina specialises in proven mental health strategies. Whether conducting group workshops or addressing large auditoriums, each presentation is meticulously tailored to the specific interests of the audience, guaranteeing it to be both captivating and a catalyst for change.

Images from speaker engagements in 2023. CWA, USU, PP, WWIB.

Book Katrina to speak at your event:
https://www.atfullpotential.com.au

Bonus Offer 3:
Online Psychology and Coaching

Katrina offers online learning opportunities that afford a self-paced and flexible delivery method, allowing you to enhance your mental health skills from the convenience of your home. These modules offer expanded information that is simple and engaging.

- o **Coaching** course: do you want to achieve your goals? This program is for 3 months and will support you to achieve your desired goals.
- o If you feel **anxiety** is preventing you from experiencing life to its fullest, successful treatment options are available. Knowing which anxiety type you have (and it is common to have more than one) will help you get the correct treatment and back in charge of your life.
- o Would you like to improve your **assertive communication**?
- o How to improve your **thinking**: what the experts know, using cutting edge brain scans to help you maintain good mental health.
- o Would you like to feel more confident about **solving problems**?
- o This module allows you to choose out of a range of different **depression** treatment options, using evidence-based therapies that fit your style.
- o If you have repeated patterns in your life that seem dysfunctional but can't quite work out why? **Schema** therapy may be able to shed light on how to make changes by first undertaking a Schema assessment.
- o **Mindfulness**: how to achieve relaxation in an ever-increasing busy world.
- o **Stress** can cause a range of health issues, learning to manage stress can have astounding benefits to your physical health and quality of life.
- o Managing your **anger** not only has significant health benefits for your but

o   If you would like to resolve **conflicts** respectfully whilst still getting your needs met, then this module has scientifically researched techniques for a range of relationships that conflicts can arise in.

o   Achieving good mental health is the ultimate goal and **preventing future relapses** is essential. This module can help you put early intervention plans in place to minimise the impact and severity of any future problems or relapses.

Look out for more book titles coming soon specifically on:

- Anxiety
- Depression
- Schema

Go to https://www.atfullpotential.com.au
and click on the link for
Online Psychology and Coaching options.

Notes